COVID-19

▼

THE
CONSPIRACY
THEORIES

COVID-19

THE CONSPIRACY THEORIES

**The truth and what's
been hidden from us**

David Gardner

jb

Published by John Blake Publishing,
an imprint of Bonnier Books UK
4th Floor, Victoria House
Bloomsbury Square
London, WC1B 4DA

Owned by Bonnier Books
Sveavägen 56, Stockholm, Sweden

www.facebook.com/johnblakebooks
twitter.com/jblakebooks

Paperback: 9781789466225
Ebook: 9781789466232
Audio: 9781789466348

A catalogue record for this book is available from the British Library.

Design by www.envydesign.co.uk

Printed and bound in Great Britain by Clays Ltd, Elcograf S.p.A

1 3 5 7 9 10 8 6 4 2

Every... ...been made to trace... ...f material
reproduce... ...the publishers

To my wife Michelle, whose strength and beauty know no bounds, and our children, Mickey, Jazmin and Savannah.

I also want to dedicate this book to all those around the world who died during this very real pandemic, many separated from their loved ones at the time they needed them most, and to the front-line workers who put their lives at risk to save ours.

'Keep your face always toward the sunshine, and shadows will fall behind you.'

Walt Whitman

INTRODUCTION

Conspiracy theories are not new. Jonathan Swift wrote over 300 years ago that 'falsehood flies, and truth comes limping after it, so that when men come to be undeceived, it is too late; the jest is over, and the tale hath had its effect.' Wars have been fought over them, they cost six million lives in the Holocaust and trust in our institutions has been shaken in defining historic events from the moon landings to JFK's assassination and 9/11.

But the global coronavirus pandemic was the perfect storm for conspiracy theories with social media fanning the flames faster and further than even Swift's vivid imagination could ever have conceived.

Like a virus, conspiracy theories have seeped so stealthily into our conversation that it's hard to tell where they started. And like a virus, they can be deadly if left to run amok.

Once upon a time, gossip and speculation would be confined to the pub or the hair salon. In the internet age, these theories can spread around the world in a matter of moments. There are few fact-checkers, fewer censors and sometimes no common sense. But theories are taken as facts and the wilder they are, the more attractive they can be to an audience that feels it is being lied to at every turn by the people they have elected to govern.

So, when COVID-19 entered the public consciousness early in 2020, first in China and inexorably through the rest of the world, it quickly became the subject of the most virulent outbreak of conspiracy theories we have ever seen. The pandemic quickly became an infodemic.

And these theorists are not all the bonkers cultists and mavericks the label is often associated with. They are your parents, your next-door neighbour, your boss at work. The question marks over the origins of COVID-19, the dangers of the virus and the best ways of treating it are the water cooler conversation of 2022, albeit many of these chats have been online from our home workspaces.

The President of the United States championed bleach as a cure, the Chinese government blamed the Americans, and the American government blamed the Chinese – a Cold War over a cold virus. People blamed 5G phone networks, genetically modified crops, Bill Gates ... aliens.

One of the biggest online battlegrounds has been over Wuhan, the ground zero of the pandemic. Was it bats or is that just bats? Was it a biological weapon accidentally (or not) unleashed on an unsuspecting planet? According to Pew Research, nearly three in ten Americans believe that COVID-19 was made in a lab and most of those think it was intentionally leaked. The very thought of such an idea was dismissed as an inflammatory conspiracy theory – until President Joe Biden ordered an investigation into those very same claims and an

American firm had to explain why it kept its findings on bat research secret.

The COVID fallout has become political and polarising with the right wing affronted by the attack on personal freedoms and the left backed into a corner on defending mandatory restrictions worthy of a fascist dictatorship.

David Icke argues COVID is a hoax and, incidentally, so did the gentleman in tweed at our Cornwall holiday hotel last summer who said he worked 'somewhere in Whitehall' and didn't believe the hospitals were full of patients. 'Do you know anyone who died?' he asked. 'Thought so.' He genuinely believed the pandemic was dreamed up by politicians intent on injecting digital markers via vaccines to keep tabs on the populace.

As with my book, *9/11: The Conspiracy Theories*, I will examine the conspiracy theories that have become as familiar to us as lockdowns, face masks and social distancing and offer a studied account of which ones are plain crazy, which are plausible and which have been covered up. With the COVID pandemic the purveyors of the conspiracy theories included governments – the people we put in power to lead us through catastrophic events such as this – and often it has been the individuals who were simply trying to understand how such a devastating virus could be allowed to run amok irrespective of borders, language, age or creed, and how best to stop it spreading. Journalists, often the truth seekers we rely on to navigate through the self-interest of politicians, found themselves being politicised to such a degree that they couldn't see the wood for the trees.

On too many levels during the pandemic, the people were left to work it out for themselves. Believing the wrong politician, the wrong theory, could kill you. And it did. A sizeable proportion of the more than six million people who have died so far from

COVID-19 could have been saved. They were misled and misinformed and the price for believing the wrong theory or the wrong person was disproportionately high.

The concept of conspiracy theories, at its essence, is about getting to the truth, not about spreading lies. With first-hand reporting and detailed investigations into the people who originated these COVID conspiracy theories, I will endeavour to answer the questions that everyone has been asking since the pandemic began and left us doubting our leaders as never before.

This is not just a book for people fascinated by conspiracy theories. This one's for all of us.

Here for the first time is the story behind the stories about the pandemic that hit the Earth like a bat out of hell.

CHAPTER 1:

TO THE BATCAVE
– 25 April 2012

▼

It was a disgusting job. The stench was overpowering as the floor was inches thick with faeces from the bats that darted through the darkness above his head in the airless mineshaft 150 feet below the earth. Rats and shrews scuttled around his feet and, although he'd been down there before, he could never quite get used to the fluttering of tiny wings in the blackness.

But Lu was a miner and, like miners everywhere, he was aware of the dangers when he ventured underground to put food on the table for his family. Besides, he was forty-two and lived close to the abandoned copper mine in the verdant hills south of the village of Tongguan in China's Yunnan province. When he was asked, along with five fellow miners, to clean up the bat guano from the abandoned cave it brought with it the promise of reopening the mine and more work for his community.

It's a region of south-west China with stark contrasts; lush vegetation where wild Asian elephants wander freely through the dense bamboo and gold and copper mines are hammered into the mountainous landscape. It's warm year-round with downpours a part of daily life, even in the driest month of February, and famous for its fermented Pu'er tea. Further north in Yunnan Province is Shangri-La, the 'lost paradise' with its fabled mirror lake, flower-strewn wetlands, Tibetan monastery and the timeless, natural beauty of fairy tales.

None of that much mattered as Lu joined three other miners on 2 April 2012, to begin clearing up the thick carpet of pellets on the Tongguan copper stream. They ignored the bats roosting above them and got to work on gruelling seven-hour shifts, the air fetid with foul-smelling faeces.

Lu was born in Zhao Tong, one of China's poorest prefectures in the north-east corner of Yunnan where temperatures frequently drop below zero on winter nights and mining is one of the dominant industries. Jobs there are scarce and the Chinese authorities encourage young people to look elsewhere for employment. Lu had worked in this mineshaft before and wasn't unduly worried at first when he developed a cough. It came with the territory.

But on around 11 April 2012, he woke with a roaring fever of around 38.5 Celsius. Occasionally, when he coughed, he noticed blood clots in the rusty-coloured mucus. He carried on working for another five days, feeling worse all the time. By 16 April, as much as he needed the work, he couldn't face going back down the mine; he lost his appetite, felt bloated in the stomach and couldn't help an uncomfortable hiccup. A blood transfusion suggested by his doctor did little to alleviate the symptoms and he was transferred to the Yu Xi People's Hospital for inpatient treatment when his temperature rose to 40 degrees Celsius. Despite the best efforts of the medical staff, Lu's condition became worse. For the next three days he struggled to breathe, especially when he tried to walk around. His only relief was lying on his back. He had no history of high blood pressure, heart disease, allergies or diabetes. Unable to stabilise the increasingly distressed miner, his doctors sent Lu to the First Established Hospital of Kunming Medical University in the province's capital about 360 kilometres from Tongguan. On 25 April 2012, Lu was carried on a stretcher into the emergency department of the hospital dominating the skyline of the ancient capital known as the 'city of eternal spring' because of its mild – healthy – climate. Ominously, Lu's lung could be heard crackling as he tried to breathe. A CT scan showed that severe pneumonia had set into his right lung. Now he was bedridden and breathing with the use of a ventilator. Lu's condition was deteriorating daily and there was nothing anyone could do.

Lu was the first of the six miners to be admitted to Kunming Medical University's First Affiliated Hospital, but he was by no means in the worst state. An older miner, Khou, sixty-three, had worked for the same amount of time in the shaft as Lu but waited an additional day before he checked in on 26 April 2012 with a raging fever. For the previous ten days Khou had been coughing, struggling to breathe, suffering chest pains and having recurring hiccups. He had checked into a local hospital in Mojiang but he was sent to Kunming once they knew Lu was under the university hospital's care in the hope they could find some answers.

Khou said he was lethargic, couldn't sleep and lost his appetite. His chest pains were getting more severe. He had been fit for his age but couldn't walk to the ward when he was admitted; a stretcher was called. Dry cackles could be heard coming from his lungs as he fought for breath. His doctors described the disease wracking Zhou's body as acute and fierce, and it seemed his ability to fight the virus was hampered by a pre-existing condition – a tumour – that left his immune system weak and vulnerable.

Later that same day, a third miner, Liu, forty-six, was rushed into the Dunming hospital's emergency room with similar symptoms, if not quite so bad. His fever hadn't broken in ten days but, although he was having difficulties with his breathing, he wasn't suffering any chest pains. Nevertheless, there was a moist crackling sound from both the lower parts of his lungs. He told the doctors he had always been very healthy.

The following day – 27 April 2012 – brought the admission of the fourth miner who had been clearing bat guano from that same cave. Guo, forty-five, was one of the four-man team with Lu, Liu and Zhou, who were initially given the task of cleaning up the mineshaft. For the previous two weeks, he, too, had been fighting a bad cough, shortness of breath and fever. In addition, he'd been coughing up yellow and greenish mucus two or three times a day. His head was banging and he complained of soreness in his limbs. Guo rallied at first, but quickly went back downhill.

Now all four miners were fighting for their lives on ventilators with their doctors racing against time to try and discover what caused their matching – and potentially deadly – symptoms.

Two younger men had been drafted in to help the bat poop clean-up when the older miners fell sick. Wu, thirty, had been working in the cave for just four days when he became ill with similar symptoms to the others – coughing, shortness of breath, mucus and fever – and was admitted to hospital on 2 May 2012. Li, thirty-two, had started working in the mine on 22 April after the others got sick and was also admitted into hospital just four days later with the same symptoms. Their conditions were not as bad as the older men, but it was clear there was a pattern – and it led back to the bat cave.

For the next month or so, the medical team's efforts were focused on keeping their patients alive even as the older men spiralled. They suspected funguses from the cave, a source of occasional medical problems in Yunnan in the past, may have been the cause.

When Zhou, the oldest and sickest of the miners, died on 7 May after twelve days in hospital, the diagnosis was:

Severe lung infection

Sepsis

Septic shock and infection in abdominal cavity

Asystole and stop breathing

'Discharge reason: death,' read the medical report.

Lu died on 12 June, forty-eight days after first raising the alarm about the bat nightmare in the mineshaft and had a slightly different discharge diagnosis, although the tragic outcome was the same:

Asystole and stop breathing

Severe pneumonia

Type 1 respiratory failure

Sepsis

Hepatitis B

Guo fought for 109 days before finally succumbing on 13 August after his crippled immune system was overwhelmed with a hospital-acquired infection. His discharge diagnosis read:

Severe pneumonia

Multiple organs failure

ARDS (Acute Respiratory Distress Syndrome)

Inhaling lung impairment

Interstitial pneumonia (virus related)

Invasive pulmonary aspergillosis

On 19 June, Professor Zhong Nanshan, a British-educated respiratory expert from The First Affiliated Hospital at Sun Yat-sen University and a former president of China's medical association who had led the country's battle with SARS-related diseases, sat in on a progress meeting remotely and suggested a visit to the Animal Laboratory at the Kunming Institute of Zoology to confirm the species of the bats in the cave and for the case doctors to conduct a swab test and Severe Acute Respiratory Syndrome (SARS) antibody examinations. It was the first suggestion that the men could have contracted a new strain of SARS-like coronavirus with the bats as the likely culprit.

The pathology examinations in the wake of the deaths were hampered by the refusal of relatives to allow autopsies to be carried out on their loved ones. They even said no to blood samples being taken.

The three other men finally recovered after suffering similar symptoms as the older miners. Liu had been in the cave for as long as his colleagues who died but managed to pull through by the skin of his teeth after spending 107 days in hospital. The other two, aged thirty and thirty-two respectively, were younger, stronger and had spent less time in the cave. They were discharged alive after twenty-six days and twenty-four days.

At Professor Zhong's suggestion, doctors sought the opinion of experts at the Kunming Institute of Zoology, who found the six miners had been exposed to the 'Chinese rufous horseshoe bat'. This conclusion left the doctors with a dilemma. All the medical and circumstantial evidence led them to believe that the bats were to blame. The six miners worked in the cave cleaning up bats' faeces. They dug it up, they breathed it in, seven hours a day, and they all suffered the same symptoms with escalating seriousness depending on age and wellness, but just seven years earlier, Shi Zhengli, head of the Wuhan Institute of Virology and one of China's most famous scientists, had published a paper in *Science* magazine insisting that SARS-like-COV viruses carried by bats was not contagious to humans.

Did this have any impact on the conclusion to a case paper on the 2012 case study written as a master's thesis by one of the doctors, Li Xu? In his report, 'The Analysis of Six Patients With Severe Pneumonia Caused by Unknown Viruses', he wrote that the condition that led to the fatal pneumonia that killed three of the miners 'could' have been 'the SARS-like-Cov from the Chinese rufous horseshoe bat or Bats kind SARS-like-Cov', rather than saying it was the definitive cause of the deaths.

As we now know, the bat virus was to blame. What Li could never have guessed was that his study would become a key piece of the jigsaw in a worldwide search for the cause of the COVID pandemic that was still puzzling scientists a decade later.

This then, is the ground zero of conspiracy theories about COVID-19. It went virtually unreported at the time. Three manual workers dying from similar symptoms as the result of working in a forgotten cave in rural China barely made a paragraph in the local press let alone the world's media. Maybe it was the result of a blackout ordered by the Chinese authorities that are paranoid about any bad publicity. Maybe there was some confusion over the possible implications. What is certainly true is that no one notified the World Health Organization, a stipulation for member states since 2007 for all 'events that may constitute a public health emergency of international concern'.

Fast-forward to the midst of a global pandemic that claimed millions of lives and left many millions more sick and vulnerable and the plight of those six miners in a Tongguan mineshaft was being dissected in Downing Street, the White House and the halls of power everywhere. The facts of the deaths are not in doubt nor, in truth, is the role the bats played in them.

But while the 2012 outbreak may have been limited to the cave workers – despite no apparent efforts to treat the cases as potentially contagious – the Wuhan Institute of Virology and Dr Zhengli, in particular, were certainly taking notice of the events in Mojiang County. To the Institute, it was an incredible opportunity to further their field-leading research into bats and they would soon be visiting the Tongguan mine to gather their own samples.

Exactly what became of those samples is still unclear. Outside investigators have been refused full access to the Wuhan lab.

China certainly has its reasons for wanting the research emanating from that cave to remain a secret, but the United States also funded experiments into the uses of the virus for its own ends. We believe and disbelieve such superpowers in equal measure. We harbour our suspicions, but we have no alternative narratives.

Depending on what you believe about the Wuhan Institute of Virology's research work on those horseshoe bat samples and the precautions it took to secure them will determine whether you agree the laboratory was blameless in causing the pandemic or that a so-called conspiracy theory that a bat virus weaponised by a lab somehow escaped to kill nearly six million people across the globe and infect more than 335 million more was not a conspiracy at all, but the truth.

The fate of the six miners was strikingly familiar to that of countless families with loved ones fighting coronavirus, with older relatives left unable to breathe and, eventually, without hope. It wasn't just the progression to pneumonia, but vascular complications such as pulmonary thromboembolism and secondary infections that tallied with later COVID-19 cases. The composite of the six miners and the comparative seriousness of their conditions was also similar. The oldest at sixty-three was the worst hit and died the fastest while the younger ones, while suffering from the symptoms, were not as bad and recovered quickly with treatment, although their immune systems remained weak for some time afterwards.

But while the virus did appear to cross to humans in the bats' lair, it didn't spread any further.

It was a very different story when COVID-19 exploded into Wuhan. No cave, no house, city or country could contain it then. How had the beast mutated into a monster?

There are 1,000 kilometres between the Tongguan mine and the Wuhan Institute of Virology. Distance is the biggest reason scientists were incredulous that the outbreak began in a city so far from China's biggest bat breeding grounds. Yunnan Province, much further south, would have made a more sensible place of origin.

But that would be forgetting the direct connection between the two places. Not long after the miners had died in anonymity, Institute scientists turned up in the cave in their Hazmat suits and protective gloves. They returned to Wuhan in 2013 with faecal samples from 276 bats – the same bats that killed the miners. Between 2015 and 2017, according to Wuhan Institute of Virology files, scientists used the bat samples in experiments to see if they could be mutated to become more infectious to humans. In simple words, they wanted to know how bats could cause a pandemic. They would soon learn in the most emphatic and horrendous terms just how they could. The big unanswered question is the role that humans played in spreading the virus so far and wide from the bat cave in Tongguan.

CHAPTER 2:

PATIENT ZERO
– 17 November 2019

▼

It was a Sunday night and curious eyes were casting skywards for a rare sighting of a Leonids meteor shower as the earth passed through a stream of cosmic debris on its journey around the sun. The celestial fireworks represented an extraordinary glimpse into the past as the human eye caught up with a comet's dusty remnants of rocks and ice that probably exploded across the planet's orbit more than a hundred years earlier.

Back on land that same evening on 17 November 2019, an unsuspecting doctor in China's Hubei Province caught sight of the future – a deadly whirlwind of death and suffering that would affect the lives of nearly every person on Earth.

The doctor was on call to treat a fifty-five-year-old man who is thought to be 'Patient Zero' – the first person to contract COVID-19.

This was six weeks before China claims that a 'cluster of pneumonia cases of unknown cause' first appeared in Wuhan, the capital of Hubei, on 31 December 2019. It wasn't until 9 January 2020 that Beijing officially declared the disease as a coronavirus outbreak to the World Health Organization.

The rest of the world had no clue what was heading their way. But Connor Reed, a Welshman working at a school in Wuhan, knew exactly what was coming.

The first British COVID patient, then twenty-five, didn't give it much thought when he woke up feeling 'a bit sniffly' on 25 November 2019, and went into work thinking he'd picked up a seasonal cold.

He would end up in hospital less than a fortnight later, barely able to breathe – all the while unaware that the city he had chosen as his home was incubating a virus that would soon be spreading around the world. His friends back home in Llandudno, worried as they were for Connor, had no reason to think that the tentacles of COVID would extend all the way to them in the space of a few months. It is those few months that are at the heart of the debate over whether the pandemic could or should have been contained.

When he woke up with the Monday morning blues on 25 November, Connor's eyes were 'a bit bleary' and he was sneezing. He thought it was a common cold, the sniffles, the kind you put up with for a while and wait for it to go away. He certainly didn't consider visiting the doctor and didn't even feel bad enough to miss work at the school in Wuhan where he had worked for the previous seven months teaching English. Well-versed in Mandarin, it wasn't like he was living in isolation in central China; he watched the news and there was nothing about viruses or any health concerns out of the ordinary. He decided it was such a mild strain he wasn't contagious and so, under the weather but otherwise unbowed, he went to work.

The next day, Connor woke with a sore throat, so he decided to get a little more proactive – he tried his mother's cure of a mug of hot water and honey. When that didn't work, he got serious and added some whiskey to the cure. Hey presto, he'd discovered the cure – a hot toddy! A very occasional drinker, Connor slept like a baby and when he woke on the fifth morning the cold had miraculously disappeared.

It was day seven when the virus hit back. He ached all over, his throat was tight, his head was thumping, his eyes were like burning coals and he had a hacking cough. He felt like crap. It was serious now. He must have the flu.

The next morning wasn't any better and Connor called in sick, saying he would probably be off for the rest of the week. The hot toddies weren't working anymore.

Connor had lost his appetite and was spending his time trying his best not to cough because it was so painful.

By day eleven, his temperature was down, and he was beginning to feel better.

By the next day, he had relapsed again. The 'flu' was back and worse than ever. In a diary published in the *Daily Mail*, Connor wrote that 'just getting up and going to the bathroom leaves me panting and exhausted.

'I'm sweating, burning up, dizzy and shivering,' he continued. 'The television is on, but I can't make sense of it. This is a nightmare. By the afternoon, I feel like I am suffocating. I have never been this ill in my life. I can't take more than sips of air and, when I breathe out, my lungs sound like a paper bag being crumpled up. This isn't right.'

He decided to see a doctor but worried about the cost of calling an ambulance. 'I'm ill, but I don't think I'm dying – am I?' he wrote in the *Mail*.

After taking his chance with a taxi, he is diagnosed with pneumonia by doctors at Zhongnan University Hospital but isn't overly concerned. He was twenty-five and healthy. He would be fine.

By day sixteen, he was in agony with his sinuses and earache, but the very worst appeared to be over and on day twenty-four, he was finally breathing normally again and had shaken off the flu-like symptoms. He even felt hungry.

Twelve days later, Connor was told by a friend that a new virus was sweeping through the city and rushed out to stock up, knowing there would be a rush on essential goods. The next day, the fears were confirmed and everyone in Wuhan was warned to stay at home.

On day fifty-two, he was officially informed that his illness was very far from a common cold – it was the 'Wuhan coronavirus'.

'Maybe I caught the coronavirus at the fish market,' Connor wrote in the *Mail*. 'It's a great place to get food on a budget, a part of the real Wuhan that ordinary Chinese people use every day, and I regularly do my shopping there. Since the outbreak became international news, I've seen hysterical reports (especially in the US media) that exotic meats such as bat and even koala are on sale at the fish market. I've never seen that. The only slightly weird sight I've seen is the whole pig and lamb carcasses for sale, with their heads on.'

Connor made headlines in the United States when the media latched onto an idea that he 'cured' COVID with hot toddies. 'I wish it had been that easy,' he wrote.

Tragically, months after his diary was published in the *Daily Mail*, Connor was found dead in the halls of residence at Bangor University in Wales, where he had returned to study for a Chinese language degree. He reportedly had drugs in his system and his mother, Hayley, told the *Sun* that he never fully recovered from his COVID ordeal and being forced to spend over twenty weeks under a harsh Chinese lockdown in Wuhan. The 17 November date for 'Patient Zero' comes from Chinese government data seen by Hong Kong's *South China Morning Post*, and, while it has not been officially confirmed, is generally believed to be the first case in the pandemic. Five new cases a day were reported each day after that until 27 December, when Dr Zhang Jixian, from Hubei Provincial Hospital of Integrated Chinese and Western Medicine, told China's health chiefs that a new coronavirus was behind the outbreak and more than 180 people were infected. By 1 January 2020, the cases had risen to 381, according to the data. The first nine cases reported in November, four men and five women, were all aged between thirty-nine and seventy-nine but none have ever been named and it's not clear whether they were all living in Wuhan at the time. Some people believe COVID-19 may have been rampant in Wuhan even earlier. Leaked medical records reportedly suggest the first case could date back as far as 25 September 2019, and show that forty patients suffering from a mysterious SARS-like pneumonia were being treated at eight hospitals between the end of September and the beginning of December and at least eight of them died.

The American-based publication *Epoch Times*, which claims to have obtained the medical files, named its 'Patient Zero' as Xiao Xgui, who was treated at the Wuhan Puren Riverside Hospital, although it should be noted that the far-right publication has strong ties to the Falun Gong religious group and is fiercely anti-Chinese.

Of course, suspected COVID cases does not mean all these patients definitely had COVID-19. There was certainly no reason for Chinese scientists to link the worrying outbreak with a bunch of miners who died in a bat-infested cave 1,000 miles away seven years earlier. But with such a dearth of reliable information about the most basic of facts, how on earth are we supposed to trust the Chinese to help prevent such a thing from ever happening again?

It's a glaring example of why so many conspiracy theories have grown up around the source of the virus – essentially scientists, governments, amateur sleuths all trying to puzzle out the pieces.

But it leads you to conclude that the Chinese must have something to hide.

It would be more than a year later, on 18 March 2021, that American scientists would offer scientific evidence that the SARS-CoV-2 virus was 'likely circulating undetected for at most two months before the first human cases of COVID-19 were described in Wuhan, China in late-December 2019'.

What was even more interesting was that they claimed the simulations they used in the study suggested that the mutating virus dies out naturally more than three-quarters of the time without causing an epidemic, much less a pandemic.

The big question that remained unanswered was what could have been done to the virus to make it so deadly? Researchers at the University of California San Diego School of Medicine and the University of Arizona used molecular dating tools and epidemiological simulations to try and work out the timing of the first COVID case. They used a 'molecular clock' technique to try and put a time on the first showing of the virus by intersecting the common number of genetic mutations and that of the common ancestor of SARS-CoV-2 and its variants. Although this method is not universally reliable, the study estimated the new coronavirus's emergence at around mid-November 2019. The report, published in the 18 March 2021 issue of *Science*, put the median number of infections at less than one before 4 November, rising to four thirteen days later and nine on 1 December. Officially, the first COVID-19 hospitalisations weren't until mid-December. The epidemic simulations based on the virus's known characteristics, such as transmissibility, showed that in 29.7 per cent of simulations the virus created self-sustaining epidemics but for the other 70.3 per cent, the virus faded away after a handful of infections in the space of, on average, just eight days. 'Our study was designed to answer the question of how long could SARS-CoV-2 have circulated in China before it was discovered,' said the report's senior author Joel O. Wertheim, PhD, associate professor in the Division of Infectious Diseases and Global Public Health at UC San Diego School of Medicine. 'To answer this question, we combined three important pieces of information: a detailed understanding of how SARS-CoV-2 spread in Wuhan before the lockdown, the genetic diversity of the virus in China and reports of the earliest cases of COVID-19 in China. By combining these disparate lines of evidence, we were able to put an upper limit of mid-October 2019 for when SARS-CoV-2 started circulating in Hubei province.'

'Typically, scientists use the viral genetic diversity to get the timing of when a virus started to spread,' said Wertheim. 'Our study added a crucial layer on top of this approach by modelling how long the virus could have circulated before giving rise to the observed genetic diversity.

'Our approach yielded some surprising results. We saw that over two-thirds of the epidemics we attempted to simulate went extinct. That means that if we could go back in time and repeat 2019 one hundred times, two out of three times, COVID-19 would have fizzled out on its own without igniting a pandemic.

This finding supports the notion that humans are constantly being bombarded with zoonotic pathogens.'

If the outbreak happened in a rural area with a much less dense population, the simulations suggested the epidemics would have petered out 94.5 per cent to 99.6 per cent of the time, perhaps offering a clue to why the mini outbreak in the isolated Yunnan cave didn't spread.

'Pandemic surveillance wasn't prepared for a virus like SARS-CoV-2,' said Wertheim. 'We were looking for the next SARS or MERS, something that killed people at a high rate, but in hindsight, we see how a highly transmissible virus with a modest mortality rate can also lay the world low.'

The world would soon learn just what damage the new coronavirus could do. It would be left guessing whether the virology experts in Wuhan trying to keep a lid on the looming disaster were their saviours – or the ones to blame for letting the killer gene genie out of the bottle.

CHAPTER 3:

THE BAT WOMAN
– 30 December 2019

The words sent a shudder through Shi Zhengli after she was called from a conference in Shanghai at just after 7pm on Monday, 30 December 2019, to take an urgent call from her boss at the Wuhan Institute of Virology. She had long been the Cassandra warning of an impending pandemic to a largely unlistening world and now her worst fears appeared to be coming true. People were falling like flies from a mysterious sickness just a stone's throw from the Institute and she was needed desperately to return and lead the search to find the cause. It wasn't just that Shi was worried about the outbreak threatening the central Chinese city, she couldn't ignore a nagging doubt that the new coronavirus detected in two Wuhan hospital patients could possibly have emanated from her lab. She knew immediately about the possible implications, if the type of virus was confirmed; it belonged to the same family that caused the twenty-first century's first and, at that time, worst SARS epidemic, killing 774 people and infecting over 8,000 in twenty-nine different countries between 2002 and 2003.

'Could they have come from our lab?' she remembers thinking as her fears came crowding in.

'Drop whatever you are doing and deal with it now,' the Institute director told her.

It took Shi and her team less than a week to connect the contagion to the virus that became known in scientific circles as SARS-CoV-2, the successor to the SARS-CoV-1 behind the 2002–03 outbreak. By then, the virus was already spreading like wildfire, initially known to the public under the more generic term coronavirus and later as COVID-19. The virus is SARS-CoV-2 and the disease it causes is COVID-19.

Shi became known as China's 'Bat Woman' and was perhaps the country's most recognisable scientist after exhaustively tracking down clues in deep, rocky caves around Nanning, the capital of Guangxi, that targeted bats as the originators of SARS, which was first identified in Foshan in China's Guangdong Province bordering Hong Kong in November 2002.

Bats, it turned out, provided a viral melting pot for coronavirus with a set of unique characteristics that enabled contagions to make the species leap across to humans and mutate to evolve into a new pathogen. They had the potential, Shi surmised, to spawn a pandemic the likes of which the world had never seen.

Bats are the only mammal capable of flight and represent one fifth of all mammals on Earth. They are also one of the oldest species, dating back fifty-two million years. Scientists describe their relationship with coronavirus as an evolutionary arms race with the virus constantly evolving to overcome the bats' highly developed immune systems which then adapt accordingly. The result is that the bat builds up antibodies and isn't in the least affected by the coronavirus it hosts and that can ultimately hook into human cells and cause such damage.

Shi and her colleagues were at Shitou Cave outside Kunming in Yunnan as part of a five-year-long field study on bat-borne viruses when they heard about the outbreak involving the miners at the Mojiang mine. They spent the next year taking samples from bats, throwing nets around the entrance every evening at dusk and waiting for the nocturnal animals to head out to feed at night. They would take saliva and blood samples and faecal swabs from the live bats and collect urine and guano pellets from the cave floor.

'The mine shaft stunk like hell,' Shi told *Scientific American*. 'Bat guano, covered in fungus, littered the cave.'

At the time, she put the miners' deaths down to fungal infections – a remark that would provoke scrutiny later – but her team did discover horseshoe bats and five other bat species in the cave with a 'high frequency of infection by a diverse group of coronaviruses'.

They found one new strain of SARS-like coronavirus and, in a report published by Shi and her colleagues in February 2016 – 'Coexistence of multiple coronaviruses in several bat colonies in an abandoned mineshaft' – it emerged that all six bat species showed coronavirus co-infection. In other words, a single animal had multiple infections, 'a phenomenon that fosters recombination and promotes the emergence of novel virus strains', the report adds. Bats were, as *Scientific American* described them, 'a flying factory for new viruses'.

In December 2019, Shi was still on the train back from her aborted conference in Shanghai as she huddled with colleagues to come up with the best tests to quickly identify the contagion. They settled on a technique called polymerase chain reaction, which amplifies the genetic material of a virus to detect its presence. Genetic sequences from coronaviruses were found in samples from five of the seven patients hospitalised in Wuhan (six of them sellers or delivery men from Wuhan seafood market) and by the end of the first week in January they had identified the virus behind the outbreak as SARS-CoV-2.

According to *Scientific American*, the genomic sequence of the virus was 96.2 per cent identical to a coronavirus the researchers had identified in horseshoe bats in Yunnan.

In a report published by Shi and her team on 3 February 2020, just as the pandemic was starting to take hold, they identify the new virus as '2019-nCoV'. Eight days later, the WHO director-general Dr Tedros Adhanom Ghebreyesus officially named the disease COVID-19.

Shi's report – A Pneumonia Outbreak Associated with a New Coronavirus of Probable Bat Origin – identifies the horseshoe bat coronavirus from the mine as 'BatCoV RaTG13'.

'The close phylogenetic relationship to RaTG13 provides evidence that 2019-nCoV may have originated in bats,' the study adds.

While Shi and the Institute scientists worked around the clock on the origins of the pandemic, the 'Bat Woman' used any spare time she had to go through her own records to check for any suspicion that samples may have been mishandled or incorrectly disposed of. Critically, she wanted to know if the genomic sequences of any of her cave samples matched those of the newly named COVID-19 virus.

She told *Scientific American* that there were no matches. 'That really took a load off my mind,' she said. 'I had not slept a wink for days.'

But if she thought that was the end of the matter, Shi was very wrong. It was just the beginning.

CHAPTER 4:

... AND ROBIN
– 10 December 2019

▼

If Shi Zhengli is China's 'Bat Woman' then surely Tian Junhua must be its 'Robin'. The father of two also works in Wuhan as the Associate Chief Technician at the Department of Disinfection and Pest Control. His laboratory at the Wuhan Municipal Center for Disease Control and Prevention (CDC) was just 700 metres from the now-closed Seafood Wholesale Market that, according to the official narrative, was the origin of the pandemic.

There is no suggestion that Tian is in any way responsible for leaking a virus that inflicted such pain and pandemonium upon the world, but he has been way more forthcoming than his more famous colleague in detailing the perils of a bat hunter and the lax precautions against infection that can sometimes happen during long trips in the wild.

In a 2017 interview with the *Wuhan Evening News*, distributed online by the Chinese state-run news agency Xinhua, the virologist admits that bat urine once 'dripped on him like raindrops' after he forgot to take security precautions during a field trip when he set off fireworks with a sky cannon to frighten the bats out of a cave and fly into a net set out to catch them at night in the Huangpi District outside Wuhan.

On several other occasions, he says bat blood was sprayed directly on to his skin when he wasn't wearing sufficient protective clothing.

Tian insists that despite isolating from his family, he was never infected by the bats but as the search for the cause of COVID-19 heated up, he faced scrutiny over just how secure the handling of coronavirus-carrier bats had been in the months and years leading up to the pandemic. Inevitably, those questions raised the spectre of a scientist unwittingly allowing the killer virus to escape from a lab.

Tian started work at the CDC after graduating from Huazhong Agricultural University, where he majored in plant protection, in 2004. In an excerpt from the *Wuhan Evening News* article, he describes how he hunted for bats with the help of his wife, despite knowing 'zero' about the creatures when he started in 2012.

'There are a large number of unknown viruses in bats, and the more thorough the study of them, the more beneficial it will be to maintain human health,' he told the outlet.

The article, translated into English from Chinese, continues:

In 2012, Tian Junhua started research on bats, and the environment for collecting bat samples was extremely harsh. The bat cave smells bad, and it is extremely dangerous on the cliffs; bats carry a lot of viruses, and there is a risk of infection if they are not careful.

In addition to knowing about bats in books, Tian Junhua's knowledge of bats can be said to be almost zero.

But he was not afraid, and took his wife to the mountains to catch bats.

'I needed help at the time. My wife and I are a professional, so she came to the Batcave with me. When others were spending their time, we were catching bats in the Batcave. It was really hard for her. I am especially grateful to her understanding and support.'

The bats are motionless during the day and cannot be caught, so Tian Junhua chose to deploy the net at night. It is extremely dangerous to enter and exit the bat cave on the cliff at night, and the bats are automatically detected by ultrasonic waves, so it is not easy to capture. Tian Junhua spent a lot of effort, squatting and guarding for several days, but he didn't catch a single one.

After trying various methods, Tian Junhua finally found that the most bats were caught by using the sky cannon, using the fireworks and sounds to alert the bats to move, and then pulling the net.

But during the operation, Tian Junhua forgot to take protective measures. Bat urine dripped on him like raindrops from the top of his head. If he was infected, he could not even find the medicine. Tian Junhua tried his best to calm himself down: 'As long as the 14-day incubation period does not cause the disease, he will be lucky to escape.' After returning home, he took the initiative to keep a distance from his wife and children and isolate for half a month. Take a breath.

The wings of bats carry sharp claws, and clips are needed when grasping bats. Big bats are prone to spurting blood after being pinched; bat blood was sprayed directly on Tian Junhua's skin several times. If infected, the consequences would be disastrous. But Tian Junhua didn't flinch at all. Fortunately, he escaped the infection.

With super perseverance, Tian Junhua captured nearly 10,000 bats, and then devoted himself to the laboratory to study these bat samples. In 2012, Tian Junhua discovered a virus in bat samples collected by Huangpi, and named it 'Huangpi virus'. The research report was published on the cover of the internationally renowned academic journal *PloS Etiology* in 2013, causing a sensation.

'Compared with the later research that relies on advanced technology and instruments, the early arrest work mainly relies on manpower, so it will be more difficult and lonely.'

The collection and identification of most research samples is the most important preliminary work, and it is also a job that many academic researchers are reluctant to touch. 'But I enjoy it and will stick to it.'

The *Washington Post* seized on a video featuring Tian that was made by the China Science Communication, a website run by the nation's Association for Science and Technology, and released on 10 December 2019, just weeks before the outbreak began to take hold.

In the glossy seven-minute film, Tian suggests that he and fellow researchers lived for several days at a time in the bat caves in their mission to catch samples. 'If our skin is exposed, it can easily come in contact with bat excrement and contaminated matter, which means this is quite risky,' he says.

'We have to live for several days in the cave,' he adds. 'There's no cellphone signal, no supplies. I can feel the fear, fear of infections, fear of getting lost. With this fear, I take every step extremely cautiously. The more I feel the fear, the more I take caution in doing the details nicely because when you find the viruses you are also most easily exposed to the viruses.'

Tian's voiceover is heard as the camera shows him in a cave without a mask or any kind of face covering while he appears to handle a vial with a sample of some kind. Moments later, Tian is seen handling a squirming bat wearing gloves, but his wrists are clearly exposed. He then uses a pair of tweezers to remove a tick from the captured bat, saying: 'This is an *Ixodes vespertilionis*. A very special type of tick. You cannot find it anywhere else.'

Still in the cave, holding the tick sample up to the light, Tian is wearing goggles but no covering over his nose or mouth as he says: 'Nothing ventured, nothing gained. It's a great day.'

It should be noted that while there has been no evidence of any lab leak at the CDC, it did move its lab to a new location near the Huanan wet market on 2 December 2019. It was days later that the first cases of contagion started to be reported at the city's hospitals. As the World Health Organization pointed out in its report on the origins of the pandemic: 'Such moves can be disruptive for the operations of any laboratory.'

The report, released in March 2021, adds: 'The Wuhan CDC lab which moved on 2nd December 2019 reported no disruptions or incidents caused by the move. They also reported no storage nor laboratory activities on CoVs or other bat viruses preceding the outbreak.'

That statement seems to be a direct contradiction of Tian's remarks in the government-sponsored video.

In the film, he says: 'It is while discovering new viruses that we are most at risk of infection.'

While the 'Bat Woman' was wary of publicity, offering

very few interviews, 'Robin' appears to have revelled in the opportunity to show off his bat-hunting adventures.

He is seen striding through bucolic countryside, net in hand, or starring in dramatic footage taken inside striking-looking caves. 'I am not a doctor, but I work to cure and save people. I am not a soldier, but I work to safeguard an invisible national defence line,' he says, adding: 'The mountains and plains serve as my office and caves are my work bench. The forest lands are my labs. But the living environment of some vectors are extremely harsh for humankind and pose a great trial.

'Wet, dark and lonely, bats usually live in caves humans can hardly reach. Only in these places can we find the most ideal virus vector samples.

'Watch out,' he tells a colleague, 'Most bats living here are horseshoe bats and Pipistrellus abramus.' Horseshoe bats, I should remind you, were deemed to be the source of the 2012 mineshaft contagion.

'If we keep our skin bare, we can easily get contact with the faeces of bats which contaminate everything,' Tian explains. 'So, it is highly risky here. It usually takes several days living in the bats' caves to analyse the symbiotic relationship between the bat population and the viruses. This is a true battle without smoke or gunpowder. This is a road never travelled, just like the caves frequented by the bats.' In the cave, again with his voice over the footage, Tian is seen making a fire with a female colleague, both wearing no protective clothing at all. If the WHO still believes the CDC wasn't working on bat viruses before the pandemic, it might like to check out Tian's quote towards the end of the mini documentary. 'In the past ten-plus years we have visited every corner of the Hubei Province, we explored dozens of undeveloped caves and studied more than

300 types of virus vectors, but I do hope these virus samples will only be preserved for scientific research,' he says, 'and will never be used in real life because humans need not only the vaccines but also the protection from the nature.' The film ends with the claim that 'nearly 2,000 types of viruses have been discovered by Chinese CDC authorities over the last twelve years.' It adds that 'only 2,284 types of virus had been discovered worldwide over the 200 years prior to China's discovery. China has taken the lead in the world in the field of Basic research of virus.' There is no doubt that China's pride in its pioneering work in virus detection has taken a battering in the wake of the COVID-19 scourge. Hindsight is a wonderful thing and Tian Junhua was clearly proud of his work and eager to show it off. The more reticent Shi Zhengli was apparently also less stringent about security in the past when hunting down her bat samples, despite telling the WHO that all scientists at the Wuhan Institute of Virology wore full protective gear. According to the *Washington Post*, Shi said in a 2018 presentation to Yixi, a Chinese TED Talks-like programme, that 'in most cases, we'd wear simpler protection, and it's okay.' Her reasoning was that bat-carrier diseases couldn't infect humans directly without an intermediate host. Slides of her team – some of them without masks or gloves – showed them using nets in a cave to catch bats and sorting samples. 'Under what situation would we increase our protection?' she continued, according to a translation by the *Post*, 'For instance, when there are too many bats in the cave, and lots of dust even as you're entering,' she added. According to a 13 March 2021 tweet by US biosecurity expert Professor Richard Ebright, of Rutgers University's Waksman Institute of Microbiology, labs in Wuhan studied bat coronaviruses using just PPEs and basic Bio Safety Level standards – BSL-2 – that

'would pose very high risk of infection of field-collection, field-survey, or laboratory staff upon contact with a virus having the transmission properties of SARS-CoV-2'. In a tweet in the same thread, he added: 'For reference, BSL-2 is the biosafety level of a US dentist's office (i.e., lockable door, screened windows, sterilizer, gown and gloves).' Battle lines were being drawn. As the deaths mounted in early 2020, so did the controversy over what exactly caused the pandemic. And Bat Woman and Robin were caught in the cross-hairs.

CHAPTER 5:
THE PERSECUTED PANGOLIN
– 30 January 2020

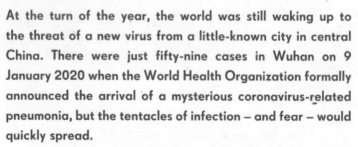

At the turn of the year, the world was still waking up to the threat of a new virus from a little-known city in central China. There were just fifty-nine cases in Wuhan on 9 January 2020 when the World Health Organization formally announced the arrival of a mysterious coronavirus-related pneumonia, but the tentacles of infection – and fear – would quickly spread.

On 20 January, three cases were reported in Japan and Thailand and the screening of passengers began at airports in Los Angeles, San Francisco and New York. The next day, a US citizen who travelled home from Wuhan to Washington became the first American with a confirmed infection and Professor Zhong Nanshan – the same expert who helped direct doctors in the 2012 mineshaft outbreak and a 1981 MD graduate from the University of Edinburgh Medical School – confirmed the disease could be spread from person to person. By the end of the month, the first two British cases of COVID-19 – two Chinese nationals staying in York – had been confirmed and the worldwide death toll had jumped to more than 200 with over 9,800 cases. It was officially a global health emergency and eyes were now wide open to the dangers of the pandemic and the potential threat to humanity.

Around this time, just as Wuhan was being put under an iron lockdown, *The Lancet* published a paper by Chinese scientists acknowledging the role of bats as the origin of the coronavirus and suggesting it had been passed on to humans via another animal host at the Wuhan wet market. Known as zoonotic spillover, this animal-to-human transmission is responsible for outbreaks of Ebola, SARS, West Nile and even the flu. It was a popular theory – it still is – and, to some extent, suits the needs of the Chinese authorities to blame nature rather than human or even systemic frailty. In their 30 January 2020 paper, 'Genomic Characterisation and Epidemiology of 2019 Novel Coronavirus: Implications for Virus Origins and Receptor Binding', the scientists said they worked on the DNA of samples from nine patients, eight of whom had visited the by now infamous Huanan seafood market in Wuhan (the ninth had stayed in a hotel close to the market between 23 and 27 December 2019). They argued that while bats were almost certainly the original 'reservoir' source of the new virus strain, another animal sold at the wet market 'might represent an intermediate host facilitating the emergence of the virus in humans'.

They zeroed in on the 'angiotensin-converting enzyme 2' (or 'ACE2') receptor, a protein the coronavirus could hook on to and infect a range of human cells. Present in many cells and tissues, including the heart, lungs, kidneys, liver, blood vessels and gastrointestinal tract, ACE2 is a vital part of the biochemical pathway, counteracting the activities of another protein called angiotensin II (ANG II) that increases blood pressure, inflammation and can damage blood vessel linings and hamper healing. When COVID-19 strikes, ANG II can inflame and kill off cells in the alveoli cells in the lungs that are critical in bringing oxygen into the body. If the coronavirus hooks into or binds to ACE2, it can no longer do its job and the ANG II is left to do its worst, often damaging the lungs and heart of COVID patients. While pointing a finger of blame at the animal market – the paper concedes that the speed of the transmissions was especially fast and that bats were almost certainly the origin – no bats were sold or found at the animal market and the outbreak was first reported in December when most bats were hibernating. Nevertheless, harking back to similar previous outbreaks when palm civets (a mongoose-type creature native to South and South East Asia) carried the virus in the SARS 2003 outbreak that started in China and dromedary camels were thought to be the intermediate hosts in the 2012 Middle East respiratory syndrome (MERS) infections in Jeddah, Saudi Arabia, the scientists claimed that 'based on current data, it seems likely that the 2019-nCoV causing the Wuhan outbreak might also be initially hosted by bats, and might have been transmitted to humans via currently unknown wild animal(s) sold at the Huanan seafood market. More generally,' the study concludes, 'the disease outbreak linked to 2019-nCoV again highlights the hidden virus reservoir in wild animals and their potential to occasionally spill over into human populations.' It is no great surprise that the animal market theory quickly caught on around the world even though the scientific evidence appeared largely circumstantial. The creatures traded in the market reads like something from the island of Dr Moreau, everything from a Siamese crocodile to an Amur hedgehog to a king ratsnake, a Chinese bamboo rat and a hog badger. A report by Oxford University biologists in collaboration with colleagues at China West Normal University, Nanchong, and Hubei University of Traditional Chinese Medicine, Wuhan, on sales at the wet market immediately prior to the pandemic between May 2017 and November 2019 says the animals were being sold both for food and as pets. Almost all of them 'were sold alive, caged, stacked and in poor condition'. Many of the live animals were slaughtered onsite for human consumption. Squirrels were sold as pets for twenty-five cents each. The sharp-nosed pit viper was the most expensive reptile, at $70 per kg. Animals caught through illegal poaching were confirmed to be on sale at the market, known as 'wet' because the ice and sprays used to keep the creatures alive and to wash away blood keep the market floors awash with water. Notably, the report confirms that neither bats nor pangolins were on sale at the market. Pangolins, also known as scaly anteaters, are said to be the most trafficked wild animal in the world; their scales, made from keratin, the same protein that makes fingernails and hair, are prized in Chinese medicine to treat ailments including arthritis, skin diseases and menstrual disorders. Found in subtropical and tropical forests from India and South China to South East Asia, pangolins were widely touted as the most likely intermediate host for the coronavirus to pass from bat to human. The evidence against the poor pangolin was circumstantial at best and an unfair strike against a species struggling for its own survival from a predator it simply wasn't armed to protect itself against ... humans. The amazing animals, no relation to the anteater, pose absolutely no danger to any animal other than ants and the odd colony of termites when they take its fancy. Elusive, solitary and shy with a tongue as long as their bodies, their default method of defence is to roll into a ball like an armour-plated hedgehog, which works well when faced with the jungle's fiercest predators but is little use against a man. In China, they are prized for their scales; in Africa their flesh is cooked and eaten. In America, before such things were banned, pangolin skins were made into cowboy boots. They can't catch a break and their numbers were dwindling even before some enterprising scientists discovered they were susceptible to coronaviruses. Few paid much attention when scientists from the Guangzhou governmental laboratory at the Guangzhou Zoo found fragments of coronavirus in a sample of twenty-one pangolins rescued in the province by customs officials. The animals were in a very bad way and sixteen of them quickly died, some with swollen lungs, and in their report, published in October 2019, the researchers suggested some may have perished as a result of the virus. Then, on 7 February 2020, a team from the South China Agricultural University in Guangzhou made a big deal of a press conference announcement that pangolins might be the 'missing link' and that the coronavirus found in pangolins was a 99 per cent match to the virus found in humans. It made a big splash around the world, especially after the Geneva-based Convention on International Trade in Endangered Species of Wild Fauna and Flora (CITES) issued a tweet reading '#Pangolins may have spread #coronavirus to humans'.

Other experts said the so-called smoking gun could quite likely blow up in the face of the South China Agricultural University team led by Professor Shen Yongyi. The science was suggestive rather than conclusive at best and lacked the usual review vetting process, such was the clamour for explanations about how the disease began. It turned out that the pangolins the scientists had sampled were not from Wuhan at all, but from the tragic, sick pangolins rescued in Guangzhou the previous

October. There was no clear evidence on how these pangolins died, let alone how they could have infected humans two or three months later in a city nearly 1,000 miles away.

Reuters news agency quoted Hong Kong City University veterinary medicine professor Dirk Pfeiffer as saying: 'You can only draw more definitive conclusions if you compare prevalence (of the coronavirus) between different species based on representative samples, which these almost certainly are not.' One thing is known for certain about the trafficked pangolins that were the subject of this study. It says they 'were mostly inactive and sobbing, and eventually died in custody despite exhausting rescue efforts'. Who did this to them? Yes, humans. The report on the wet market sales by the collaboration of Chinese and Oxford scientists, published in Nature.com on 7 June 2021, appeared to confirm that there weren't even any pangolins at the market.

'Circumstantially,' it says, 'the absence of pangolins (and bats, not typically eaten in Central China; media footage generally depicts Indonesia) from our comprehensive survey data corroborates that pangolins are unlikely implicated as spillover hosts in the COVID-19 outbreak. This is unsurprising because live pangolin trading has largely ceased in China.' The report warns that jumping to conclusions could be disastrous for the animals, saying: 'We should therefore not be complacent, because the original source of COVID-19 does not seem to have been established. This is doubly important because false attribution can lead to extreme and irresponsible animal persecution. For instance, civets were killed en masse following the SARS-CoV outbreak, and any unwarranted vilification or persecution of pangolins and bats in relation to COVID-19 would risk undermining otherwise very successful efforts to better protect and conserve wildlife in China.' David Macdonald,

Oxford University's first Professor of Wildlife Conservation, part of the college's Department of Zoology, was a member of the research team, and confirmed 'that both bats and pangolins had an alibi – neither was there!' In a 7 June 2021 column for the Oxford Science Blog, Professor Macdonald wrote that:

> Bats are actually rarely consumed in Central China, where market photos generally depict Indonesia. Pangolin trade is still a significant issue in other Chinese cities and trading nodes, but not in Wuhan. What were there, however, were 47,381 individuals from thirty-eight species, including thirty-one protected species, all kept in dreadful conditions and teeming with all kinds of other infectious diseases, ready to be slaughtered on demand, if not sold as pets…With these huge concentrations of diverse species under one roof, while we discovered no evidence supporting original spill-over from candidate bats or pangolins in Wuhan, it would seem but a matter of time before some other unwelcome disease might skip into the human population,' he wrote, adding: 'Indeed it is estimated that around 70 per cent of all diseases afflicting people originate in animals, think avian influenza, HIV, Ebola, etc.

The Chinese government moved swiftly as many settled on the animal market as public enemy number one in the hunt for a coronavirus culprit. On 26 January, it temporarily banned all wildlife trade and a little over a month later it made it illegal to eat and trade terrestrial wild animals. The Wuhan market was shut down, probably for ever.

China's actions were commended by Professor Macdonald,

who wrote that they would have 'collateral benefits for global biodiversity conservation and animal welfare and will hopefully prevent some future tragedies'.

All these things are true, and we can only hope that the spotlight on wet markets such as the one in Wuhan will result in better controls and more humane treatment of animals in China and elsewhere in the world in the future.

But fundamental questions about the wet market theory remained. If bats were, indeed, the source of contamination at the market, how come there were no bats to be found there? If another animal at the market was the intermediate host – the bridge between bats and humans – and it wasn't the falsely accused pangolin, then what creature was it? Wouldn't we know by now, just as we knew about the MERS camel in Saudi and the humble SARS civet after China's previous coronavirus outbreak?

And if scientists insist that the wet market represents the only logical ground zero for COVID-19 because the virus can only be transmitted from bats via another animal, are they then forgetting the three Yunnan miners killed in the abandoned mineshaft in 2012?

In November 2020, Denmark announced it had culled more than 17 million minks following coronavirus outbreaks at more than 200 mink farms across the country. Danish officials said the virus spread from human handler to the minks, mutated and passed back to humans. No mink was spared; every one of the animals famed for their luxurious fur were killed whether or not they were infected despite the fact the disease was spread by humans. If we infected the minks, is it not then possible that humans are the intermediate hosts and that the SARS civets and the MERS camels, like the poor pangolins, got a bad rap and were, in fact, framed by the real super-spreaders – the humans?

Look, I'm not ruling the Huanan Seafood Market out as the source, but if it was, wouldn't you think some verifiable evidence to prove it was the cause of the worst pandemic of the twenty-first century would have surfaced by now?

For a moment, at least, the outrage over treatment of the menagerie of weird and wonderful creatures on sale in Wuhan took the attention away from the virology labs located in the same section of the city.

But that was about to change in February 2020 when two Chinese scientists published a paper – since withdrawn – claiming that 'the killer coronavirus probably originated from a laboratory in Wuhan'.

The heat was back on Bat Woman and Robin – and it was going to get a whole lot hotter.

CHAPTER 6:

BACK TO THE BATLAB
– 6 February 2020

The report by Chinese scientists Botao Xiao and Lei Xiao was devastating in its brevity. At a little over one page, 'The possible origins of 2019-nCoV coronavirus' did not come up with any ground-breaking theories for the cause of COVID-19. But the 6 February 2020 paper, supported by the National Natural Science Foundation of China, demolished the wet market theory in seven paragraphs.

With the study was a simple diagram, showing just how close the Wuhan CDC was from the market – 277.73 metres (911.06 feet) to be exact.

The paper was a preprint, meaning it lacked the peer reviewing necessary for publication in a scientific journal. But the accompanying text didn't beat around the bush.

At that point at the beginning of February 2020, the scientists were still referring to the outbreak as an epidemic, rather than a pandemic and the known laboratory-confirmed infections in

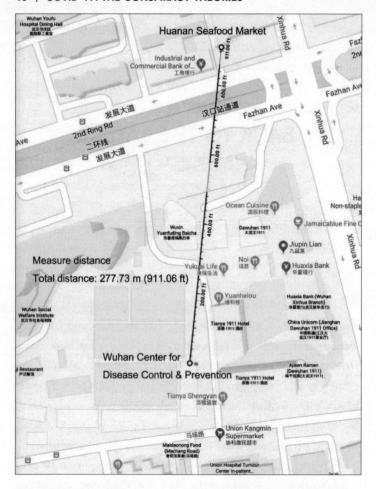

Distance from Huanan Seafood Market to Wuhan CDC (Baidu/Google Maps)

humans in China totalled 28,060, with 564 deaths. The report quoted a *Nature* article putting the genome sequences from patients at '96 per cent or 89 per cent identical to the Bat CoV ZC45 coronavirus originally found in Rhinolophus affinis'.

'It was critical to study where the pathogen came from and how it passed onto humans,' the paper continues.

Of the forty-one people in Wuhan who were afflicted,' it adds,quoting from another article in The Lancet, 'twenty-seven of them had contact with the Huanan Seafood Market.' The COVID virus was found in 33 of the 585 samples collected from the market after the outbreak, it says.

The paper questions the idea that bats would fly around the market or be sold in 'densely populated' Wuhan, a city of fiteen million people. 'The bats carrying CoV ZC45 were originally found in Yunnan or Zhejiang province, both of which were more than 900 kilometers away from the seafood market,' it says.

It also says there was little proof that the virus piggy-backed onto humans via an intermediate source.

The authors zeroed in on two laboratories conducting bat coronavirus research close to the seafood market. The first was the Wuhan Center for Disease Control & Prevention (WHCDC), which they say was within 280 metres of the market and 'hosted animals in laboratories for research purpose, one of which was specialized in pathogens collection and identification'.

'In one of their studies,' it adds, '155 bats including Rhino-lophus affinis were captured in Hubei province, and another 450 bats were captured in Zhejiang province 4.' The paper highlights the 'expert' involved in collecting the bat samples describing how he was attacked by bats and getting blood on his skin, how he quarantined himself after being contaminated with bat urine and was 'thrilled' after capturing a bat with a live tick.

'Surgery was performed on the caged animals and the tissue samples were collected for DNA and RNA extraction and sequencing. The tissue samples and contaminated rashes were source of pathogens,' the report says, adding that the WHCDC was close to the Union Hospital, where the first group of doctors were infected with COVID.

'It is plausible that the virus leaked around and some of them contaminated the initial patients in this epidemic, though solid proofs are needed in future study,' it concludes.

The authors identified the second lab as the Wuhan Institute of Virology, Chinese Academy of Sciences, saying it was twelve kilometres from the seafood market.

'This laboratory reported that the Chinese horseshoe bats were natural reservoirs for the severe acute respiratory syndrome coronavirus (SARS-CoV) which caused the 2002-3 pandemic,' it says, adding: 'The principal investigator participated in a project which generated a chimeric virus using the SARS-CoV reverse genetics system, and reported the potential for human emergence. A direct speculation was that SARS-CoV or its derivative might leak from the laboratory.'

The summary suffers a little in translation, but it clearly appears to point the finger of suspicion at the labs.

'Somebody was entangled with the evolution of 2019-nCoV coronavirus,' it says. 'In addition to origins of natural recombination and intermediate host, the killer coronavirus probably originated from a laboratory in Wuhan.'

In conclusion, the study recommends 'reinforced' safety precautions in 'high risk biohazardous laboratories' and suggests new rules 'to relocate these laboratories far away from city center and other densely populated places.'

The article was published on a site called ResearchGate. Within weeks, one of the authors, Botao Xiao, a DNA expert who was trained at America's Northwestern University, had withdrawn the paper, telling the *Wall Street Journal* in an email: 'The speculation about the possible origins in the post was based on published papers and media, and was not supported by direct proofs.'

Maybe the decision to back off from the suggestion that some kind of lab leak was the origin of the pandemic had something to do with the British tabloids picking up on the report and raising the suspicion of a cover-up.

A group of twenty-seven public health scientists from eight countries – including Sir Jeremy Farrar OBE from the UK – saw fit to sign an open letter published in *The Lancet* declaring their support for the Chinese virologists and blasting 'conspiracy theories suggesting that COVID-19 does not have a natural origin'.

'Scientists from multiple countries have published and analysed genomes of the causative agent, severe acute respiratory syndrome coronavirus 2 (SARS-CoV-2), and they overwhelmingly conclude that this coronavirus originated in wildlife, as have so many other emerging pathogens,' the letter adds.

The letter didn't pull any punches, adding: 'Conspiracy theories do nothing but create fear, rumours, and prejudice that jeopardise our global collaboration in the fight against this virus. We support the call from the Director-General of WHO to promote scientific evidence and unity over misinformation and conjecture.'

The sentiments were commendable, throwing support behind colleagues working around the clock not only to identify the causes but also to combat its catastrophic effects. Did they throw their hats into the ring a little early to know the full facts before condemning questions increasingly being asked about the reasons for China's secrecy over the fraught early days of the emerging nightmare?

Transparency is the enemy of conspiracy theories. To most thinking people, it exposes the lies and leaves a simple, clear path to the truth. Governments and those in power tend to fuel them for their own ends. Would we still be wondering what really happened on the grassy knoll in Dallas if the US government came clean on everything it knew about the John F. Kennedy assassination? Does the Royal Family know more than it has let on about the Paris car crash that killed Princess Diana? Why do so many questions about 9/11 remain more than two decades after the attacks on New York and Washington?

These are serious questions about democratic countries that pride themselves on their freedoms and open government. Why then should we be surprised when a proud and secretive nation that keeps its population in line through intimidation and has a selective sense of the truth doesn't throw open its gates and invite the world in to judge whether, by an accident of geography, by an accident or even through criminal negligence, it unleashed a deadly plague on the world?

Internal Communist Party papers reportedly seen by the Associated Press appeared to show that the country's leadership was warned about the consequences of the outbreak but delayed six days before disclosing those fears to the public. This was a crucial time. During those six days between 14 and 20 January 2020, millions of Chinese people travelled for the New Year holiday and over 3,000 contracted the virus.

At around that time, the fate of the six miners in the Yunnan mineshaft eight years earlier came back to haunt 'Bat Woman' Shi Zhengli. After several sleepless nights, she may have reassured herself and her bosses that the institute was blameless for the escalating crisis, but her team's handling of the earlier outbreak was being scrutinised.

While she had found the bats in the cave carried coronaviruses, which aligned with her acclaimed work to find the origins of the 2003 SARS epidemic, and had gone back to the scene a number of times to take 1,322 samples and build a substantial bat research lab back in Wuhan, Shi had insisted there was no evidence that SARS was the reason the three miners died. That would not have fitted in with her belief that an intermediate host was required for the virus to jump from bat to human.

From the bat samples, Shi and her colleagues had detected an astonishing 293 highly diverse coronaviruses. Of these, 284 were alphacoronaviruses and nine were designated as betacoronaviruses, which include SARS-CoV and SARS-CoV-2 (which causes the disease COVID-19).

All of the nine Yunnan bats with betacoronavirus carried SARS-related coronaviruses (SARSr-CoVs) and one of those, sample ID4991, was referred to in a 2016 report that mentioned the bats and the viruses and the fact that they were found in the Tongguan mine but made no reference to the fact that six miners fell sick and three died.

In 2018, with improving DNA technology, Shi rechecked the sequences of the bat samples, including the one numbered ID4991 which, rather confusingly, was renamed RaTG13 to reflect the type of bat (horseshoe from the Rhinolophidae affinis family), the location (Tongguan) and the year the sample was collected (2013). RaTG13 was different from the other eight samples but was not deemed to be of any great significance.

Still, Shi insisted the coronavirus-specific RdRp genes they found in the SARS-CoV bats were 'distant cousins' to the genes that led to COVID-19. RaTG13 wasn't seen as anything remarkable, and the sample was used up in testing, leaving only a sequencing memory in the lab's database.

According to the *MIT Technology Review*, it was a student on Shi's team, Si Haorui, who discovered that RaTG13 was more important than anyone had previously thought just days after the start of the outbreak. When seven of the early patients in Wuhan were tested in hospital, five of them were found to have the coronavirus RdRp genes and it was Si's job to sequence the genetic material in the patient samples to try and pin down the mysterious cause of their breathing difficulties.

When the computer analysis revealed a coronavirus, Shi checked her data banks for a possible match. Up popped sample 4991, the peculiar sequence from the bats in the mineshaft that was renamed RaTG13. It was 96 per cent identical to the coronavirus found in the first patients in the Wuhan outbreak.

Shi steadfastly maintained both that her team had not detected any coronavirus in the miners' samples they had been sent from the hospital where they were being treated in 2012 and that, while they may be related, there was a genetic gulf between the two viruses. Writing for *MIT Technology Review*, Jane Qiu – one of the few journalists to interview Shi – quotes several senior virologists supporting the 'Bat Woman'. Among them was David Robertson, a virologist at the University of Glasgow, who said: 'RaTG13 couldn't have naturally morphed into SARS-CoV-2.'

Another virologist, Angela Rasmussen, of Canada's University of Saskatchewan, said making SARS-CoV-2 from RaTG13 'would have required a feat of unprecedented genetic engineering'.

It would have helped if there was a RaTG13 sample left to test – but it was all gone.

The scientific world was split at this point and Shi remained adamant that her lab had behaved perfectly properly throughout, but there could be no independent corroboration. The Chinese wouldn't allow it. As much as the Chinese authorities tried to prevent it, the path to understanding COVID-19 remorselessly led back to that remote, abandoned mineshaft. Rather than becoming clearer over time, the road had become even murkier.

It didn't help that even the bats were now under armed guard. A checkpoint was set up on the road to the Tongguan cave and foreign journalists were prevented from going any further, on one occasion being told that rampaging wild elephants made it too dangerous to pass. When a reporter from the *Wall Street Journal* managed to reach the mine by mountain bike after hearing about the 2012 deaths, he was detained by police and held for five hours. A mobile phone picture he had snapped of the cave was deleted. Villagers said they had been told not to talk about the mine with outsiders.

The hunt for the truth was about to get politicised as never before. It wasn't just the scientists who were at odds now. Conspiracy theories about COVID-19 soon divided families, neighbours and countries and what you believed could well depend on your politics, your age or your nationality. Conflicting theories about the virus would go way beyond what caused it, but that was the beginning. If we couldn't agree on what caused the pandemic, what could we agree on?

Up to this point, the darkest speculation involved a terrible mistake, an innocent lab leak caused by carelessness or ineptitude. Suspicions about the role of RaTG13 unleashed a much more sinister theory about how the pandemic started that would send shock waves around the world and have serious consequences for Chinese nationals, especially those living in the West.

This theory wouldn't be so easy to dismiss, whatever the science and whether it was true or not – because it was being championed by the President of the United States.

CHAPTER 7:

THE BIRMINGHAM
LAB LEAK
– 25 July 1978

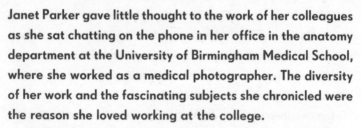

Janet Parker gave little thought to the work of her colleagues as she sat chatting on the phone in her office in the anatomy department at the University of Birmingham Medical School, where she worked as a medical photographer. The diversity of her work and the fascinating subjects she chronicled were the reason she loved working at the college.

On 25 July 1978, Parker had spent more time than usual on the phone in her dark room ordering photographic materials. It is unlikely that she knew that a new strain of smallpox was being handled that same day in a lab on the floor immediately below her. If she did, it probably wouldn't have concerned her as the university had a stellar reputation. Besides, the forty-year-old had been vaccinated against smallpox twelve years earlier.

It wasn't until 11 August that the former police photographer started to feel unwell. Her muscles began to ache and she couldn't shake off a drilling headache. At first, the spots on her skin were diagnosed as a rash and then chickenpox. By 20 August when she was admitted to East Birmingham Hospital, the spots were covering her body, including her face and the palms of her hands and the soles of her feet. She was diagnosed with smallpox and quickly transferred to an isolation hospital in nearby Solihull. That night, as the seriousness of her situation became apparent, Parker's parents and anyone she had been in touch with were rushed into quarantine.

The diagnosis was confirmed by Henry Bedson, head of the smallpox laboratory at the medical school as the finger of suspicion was pointed at a leak from his department right beneath Parker's office. He faced a trial by media and a hailstorm of controversy over the handling of smallpox samples in his lab and questions over possible genetic manipulation.

On 6 September 1978, Bedson killed himself, cutting his throat in the garden of his Birmingham home where he was quarantined. His suicide note read: 'I am sorry to have misplaced the trust which so many of my friends and colleagues have placed in me and my work.'

Parker died a painful, lonely death five days later on 11 September 1978 – the last recorded person to die of smallpox, one of history's deadliest diseases that claimed the lives of more than 300 million people since 1900 alone.

A British government inquiry into Parker's death found she had been infected by the smallpox strain being handled in the lab below and said the likeliest cause was the air ducts linking the two floors. A court later vindicated the university with experts claiming it would take twenty years for one particle to travel up to the dark room office if it escaped from the smallpox sample below.

The circumstantial evidence was certainly hard to ignore, but the truth is that nobody really knew how the photographer was infected and they still don't to this day.

An unprecedented worldwide, vaccination programme killed off the smallpox threat and in 1978 the World Health Organization was about to announce it as the first disease ever to be eradicated.

But accidents can still happen.

Swift action and vaccinations worked to limit the effects of the Birmingham smallpox outbreak, but it is far from being alone in the pantheon of pathogen lab leaks.

In 1978, rumours emerged from the Soviet Union that hundreds of people had contracted anthrax in the remote city of Sverdlovsk and the Soviets blamed it on contaminated meat. US intelligence officials disagreed, claiming a weaponised form of anthrax had been accidentally leaked from a mysterious military facility known as 'Compound 19'.

Ronald Reagan, America's president at the time, asked scientists to investigate the case and they essentially agreed with the Soviet explanation, saying it was 'completely plausible'.

It was only with the break-up of the Soviet Union that the truth became clear. Pathology samples from the victims' lungs revealed they had inhaled anthrax leaked from 'Compound 19', which turned out to be a secret bioweapons facility. Simple human error was to blame for the deaths of at least sixty people. The officer in charge had forgotten to inform the next shift that spores on the machine had become clogged – apparently a regular occurrence – and it spluttered out a deadly plume of anthrax spores when it was restarted the following morning.

Back in Britain, the 2007 foot-and-mouth outbreak that

prompted the slaughter of 600 cattle and a three-week ban on livestock exports was blamed on a virus leaking from poorly maintained drains at a lab to nearby farms.

More pertinently, since the first SARS outbreak in China in 2003 there have been at least six lab leaks involving the virus.

Scott Gottlieb, the former head of the US Food and Drug Administration (FDA), told CBS TV show *Face the Nation* that lab leaks 'happen all the time'.

'Even here in the United States, we've had mishaps,' he continued. 'And in China, the last six known outbreaks of SARS-1 have been out of labs, including the last known outbreak, which was a pretty extensive outbreak that China initially wouldn't disclose that it came out of a lab.'

The six SARS leaks happened in three countries – Singapore, Taiwan and China – with two happening in one month in a lab in Beijing and resulting in the death of the mother of a lab worker.

That the Chinese have history in prevarication is hardly a surprise. There were the strangest anomalies during the H1N1 influenza pandemic that emerged from China in 1977–78 and killed over 700,000 people around the world. For one, the victims were almost all in their mid-twenties or younger and the strain was almost identical to one from the 1950s. It also seemed that people before then had developed an immunity that the younger generations just didn't have.

Later, a senior Chinese virologist admitted that the pandemic spread after a virus frozen in the 1950s was used in 1977 vaccine trials involving thousands of military recruits. As *New York Times* columnist Zeynep Tufekci wrote on 25 June 2021: 'For the first time, science itself seemed to have caused a pandemic while trying to prepare for it.'

Referring to COVID-19, she continued: 'Now, for the second

time in fifty years, there are questions about whether we are dealing with a pandemic caused by scientific research.'

But it wasn't the idea that scientists just may have made a mistake that raised temperatures in the halls of power as the infections piled up around the world. Scientists, like politicians and journalists, hate to admit fault. Nevertheless, as we have seen, they happen all the time. Virology is a competitive business and breakthroughs bring plaudits and profits. Coming second is coming last and when you are dealing with countries like China and the United States, losing is anathema.

An accidental leak doesn't mean there was any malicious intent. It just takes a lab worker to be unwittingly exposed to a virus, go home and spread it to others.

At issue now was not just how scientists were tinkering with their coronavirus samples but why. As the first spring of COVID-19 developed into a global pandemic of nightmare proportions, there was growing disquiet over China's reticence to release all its research and data on SARS-CoV-2 and the way it was cherry-picking what information to share with the world. More specifically, there was a focus on what scientists call 'gain of function' research, a kind of genetic manipulation of micro-organisms.

Gain of function work is nothing new; scientists have been carrying out benign experiments for decades, everything from playing with enzymes to create a new type of beer to messing with a mosquito virus so it won't transmit dengue fever. These are potentially good things and there is no end of similar examples of experiments seeking new ways to positively further knowledge. Indeed, COVID-19 vaccinations from Oxford-AstraZeneca and Johnson & Johnson are based on safe adenoviruses modified to produce the spike protein for SARS-CoV-2.

But gain of function research gets on more shaky ground when it meddles with the effects of pathogens between different species.

In 2011–12, the headlines were full of the fast-mutating avian influenza virus H5N1, or 'bird flu', which killed millions of birds and was unpleasant and occasionally deadly for humans but containable, chiefly because almost everyone who caught the virus got it directly from handling birds and it wasn't transmissible from one person to another. Inevitably, there was concern at the devastation such a virus could cause if it were transmissible on a scale such as the 1918 Spanish flu that killed around fifty million people.

Scientists in the US and Holland decided to investigate what it would take to mutate the bird flu into a plague virus to better understand just how close the world was to a potential catastrophe. To do this, they took their gain of function techniques one step further from simply mutating the virus in a Petri dish to passing it through another animal rather than cell cultures. The animal they chose was a ferret, a decent enough mammal stand-in for humans. If the ferrets infected each other with the mutated virus, it was reasonable to believe that humans would do the same.

The idea was that one ferret would be infected with the bird flu and when it got sick a sample of the virus would be taken from its body and used to infect a second ferret and then a third and so on until the mutated virus had passed through ten ferrets. At that point, another ferret in a separate cage who had not been physically infected fell sick with the virus, showing it was transmissible in ferrets and, by implication, in humans. The scientists had succeeded in creating a pandemic in a lab.

When Ron Fouchier, the Dutch researcher who pioneered

the work, published details in *Science* journal, it provoked a huge backlash among scientists and politicians alike amid fears a deadly pathogen could leak from his lab. Writing in *Nature*, Harvard epidemiologist Marc Lipsitch claimed Fouchier's work, 'entails a unique risk that a laboratory accident could spark a pandemic, killing millions'.

The Dutchman was defiant, insisting: 'We need GOF experiments to demonstrate causal relationships between genes or mutations and particular biological traits of pathogens. GOF approaches are absolutely essential in infectious disease research.' His new viruses were, after all, weakened and non-lethal.

But Lipsitch and a group of top scientists from around the world formed a group called the Cambridge Working Group and issued a statement on 14 July 2014, laying out their fears that such gain of function 'laboratory creation' could be disastrous.

Recent incidents involving smallpox, anthrax and bird flu in some of the top US laboratories remind us of the fallibility of even the most secure laboratories, reinforcing the urgent need for a thorough reassessment of biosafety. Such incidents have been accelerating and have been occurring on average over twice a week with regulated pathogens in academic and government labs across the country. An accidental infection with any pathogen is concerning. But accident risks with newly created 'potential pandemic pathogens' raise grave new concerns. Laboratory creation of highly transmissible, novel strains of dangerous viruses, especially but not limited to influenza, poses substantially increased risks. An accidental infection in such a setting could trigger outbreaks that would be difficult or impossible to control. Historically, new strains of influenza, once they establish transmission in the human population, have infected a quarter or more of the world's population within two years. For any experiment, the expected net benefits should outweigh the risks. Experiments involving the creation of potential pandemic pathogens should be curtailed until there has been a quantitative, objective and credible assessment of the risks, potential benefits, and opportunities for risk mitigation, as well as comparison against safer experimental approaches. A modern version of the Asilomar process, which engaged scientists in proposing rules to manage research on recombinant DNA, could be a starting point to identify the best approaches to achieve the global public health goals of defeating pandemic disease and assuring the highest level of safety. Whenever possible, safer approaches should be pursued in preference to any approach that risks an accidental pandemic.

It was a similar type of gain of function research that Shi Zhengli and her team at the Wuhan Institute of Virology undertook with the coronavirus samples they found in the Tongguan bat cave. Shi, working with American virologists from the University of North Carolina, used the strain samples to see if they could be adapted to increase their transmissibility in humans. In 2015, they used 'cut and paste' DNA engineering to mutate its make-up with the hope of making it more transmissible. Put simply, surface proteins from the SARS-like bat coronavirus from the Yunnan cave were inserted into the original 2003 SARS, creating a mash-up virus that was able to break into human cells. Underlining how transmissible it had become, the mash-up also made mice sick.

The message was as concerning as it was prescient; coronaviruses represented an urgent threat to the human race.

While the animal passage technique pioneered in ferrets by Fouchier would be difficult to spot as it replicates a kind of evolution on acid, *Newsweek* suggested the Wuhan lab's work 'could be easily flagged in a genetic analysis, like a contemporary addition to an old Victorian house'.

There is no evidence that Shi or the Institute was working through animal passage techniques on the cave bat samples, but the *Newsweek* report asserts: 'It's possible that the work was done in secret. It's possible that it never happened at all. But some scientists think it's unlikely that an expensive BSL-4 lab would not be doing animal passage research, which by 2018 was not unusual.'

Published analysis of SARS-CoV-2 suggests that there is no evidence of tell-tale manipulation of the genetic features of the virus, claiming the spike in the protein the virus uses to attach on to and disable the body's ACE2 receptors differs from the original SARS virus and offers no indication of being mutated in a lab. In her defence, Shi Zhengli remains adamant that is the case and there is an argument that the 2015 experiment was not gain of function as the original SARS coronavirus was already transmissible to humans.

Scientific opinion is less certain about the animal passage gain of function technique and the jury is out on whether that could yet be the missing piece of the puzzle.

Still, the careful peer reviewing and methodological process that science prides itself on was all about to go out of the window.

The politicians were calling the shots now.

CHAPTER 8:
THE COLDS WAR
– 17 February 2020

The venerable *Washington Post* was in a pickle. It had used the words conspiracy theory to describe an opinion expressed by a Republican senator and hard-line supporter of President Donald Trump and now it was eating humble pie.

The headline of the *Post* story first published on 17 February 2020, read: 'Tom Cotton keeps repeating a coronavirus conspiracy theory that was already debunked'.

It was later replaced with another heading: 'Tom Cotton keeps repeating a coronavirus fringe theory that scientists have disputed'. Immediately beneath it was a correction, which read: 'Earlier versions of this story and its headline inaccurately characterised comments by Sen. Tom Cotton (R-Ark.) regarding the origins of the coronavirus. The term "debunked" and the *Post*'s use of "conspiracy theory" have been removed because, then as now, there was no determination about the origins of the virus.'

It had taken the *Post* fifteen months to publish the correction, a lifetime in the news cycle, but the debacle had touched a sensitive nerve. After all, the *Post*'s big moment – journalism's big moment – the paper's investigation into the Watergate scandal that brought down President Richard Nixon had begun life being dismissed as a conspiracy theory. Who would believe the most powerful man in the world would be behind a tawdry burglary? Time eventually told a different story.

Political partisanship was clouding the probe into the COVID-19 pandemic and the *Post* and its heavyweight media companions were finding themselves drawn into a scientific debate that had no place in politics but was taking centre stage in Washington, nevertheless.

Nobody would accuse Harvard-educated Tom Cotton of being another Woodward and Bernstein, but his so-called 'fringe theory' as the *Post* would redefine it was far from crazy. In essence, he was going public with what many scientists were thinking. In an interview with Fox News at a time when most of the world was still trying to work out what was going on and how the outbreak began, Cotton cast suspicion on the Wuhan Institute of Virology.

'We don't know where it originated, and we have to get to the bottom of that,' he said. 'We also know that just a few miles away from that food market is China's only biosafety level 4 super laboratory that researches human infectious diseases.

'Now, we don't have evidence that this disease originated there, but because of China's duplicity and dishonesty from the beginning, we need to at least ask the question to see what the evidence says. And China right now is not giving any evidence on that question at all,' he added.

In a series of tweets on 16 February, Cotton had laid out his position more carefully. 'We ought to be transparent with the

American people about all this. Maybe some of these so-called experts think they know better. I don't. And they really don't either,' he tweeted, adding: 'Again, none of these are "theories" and certainly not "conspiracy theories". They are hypotheses that ought to be studied in light of the evidence, if the Chinese Communist Party would provide it.

'Let me debunk the debunkers,' he continued, tweeting that the *Washington Post* writer 'and her "experts" wrongly jump straight to the claim that the coronavirus is an engineered bioweapon. That's not what I've said. There's at least four hypotheses about the origin of the virus.'

He went on to list the options, as he saw them:

'Natural (still the most likely, but almost certainly not from the Wuhan food market)

Good science, bad safety (e.g. they were researching things like diagnostic testing and vaccines, but an accidental breach occurred)

Bad science, bad safety (this is the engineered bioweapon hypothesis, with an accidental breach)

Deliberate release (very unlikely, but shouldn't rule out till the evidence is in)'

The *New York Times* piled in with a February 2020 story headlined, 'Senator Tom Cotton Repeats Fringe Theory of Coronavirus Origins' and included a line in the story that read: 'Although much remains unknown about the coronavirus, experts generally dismiss the idea that it was created by human hands. Scientists who have studied the coronavirus say it resembles SARS and other viruses that come from bats. While contagious, so far it appears to largely threaten the lives of older people with chronic health issues, making it a less-than-effective bioweapon.'

A report at the same time on public service station NPR, America's equivalent to the BBC, said there was 'virtually no chance' the lab theory thesis was correct.

There was undoubtedly a lot of misinformation being spread in a social media phenomenon the World Health Organization labelled an 'infodemic'.

We will look at many of these later, some of them make sense, many more were plain crazy, but the political machinations were clouding the genuine search to find the defining answer to the biggest question of all – what caused the pandemic?

Donald Trump's presidency had undoubtedly contributed to the confrontational nature of the debate. Under Trump, few issues, if any, were aired without sides being drawn and COVID-19 was never going to be one of them. The former real estate tycoon and TV reality star had paved his road to the White House with promises to go tough on China over trade and had bombarded Beijing with embargoes once he moved into the Oval Office.

Right from the outset, Trump was seeking to play down the scale of the crisis in public while apparently conceding the seriousness of the situation in private.

Speaking to the *Washington Post*'s Watergate journalist Bob Woodward on 7 February 2020, at a time when just twelve people had tested positive for the coronavirus, Trump apparently called it 'deadly stuff' and described it as being five times more lethal than even the most 'strenuous flu'.

The next week, he went on TV to say the virus was 'very mild' and told supporters at a rally not to worry because it would 'miraculously go away' when the weather warmed up in April.

He would later claim he played the pandemic down to avoid creating panic but as the numbers of deaths and infections shot up, the president hit on another tactic that would both appeal to his supporters and avoid him being fact-checked when the numbers went against him. He turned the heat up on his nemesis in Beijing.

The president repeatedly called COVID-19 the 'Chinese virus', ignoring reports of widespread abuse and violence against Chinese Americans who were wrongly blamed for spreading the disease in the early days of the pandemic.

At a White House press conference on 18 March 2020, Trump defended his use of the words, insisting: 'It's not racist at all.'

Asked why he continued to use the words Trump answered: 'Because it comes from China. That's why. I want to be accurate.'

The White House followed up with a tweet of its own to back the president, saying: 'Spanish Flu. West Nile Virus. Zika. Ebola. All named for places. Before the media's fake outrage, even CNN called it Chinese Coronavirus. Those trying to divide us must stop rooting for America to fail and give Americans real info they need to get through the crisis.'

The previous day, Chinese-born CBS News White House Correspondent Weijia Jiang tweeted: 'This morning a White House official referred to #Coronavirus as the "Kung-Flu" to my face.

'Makes me wonder what they're calling it behind my back,' added Jiang.

Secretary of State Mike Pompeo, America's number one diplomat, tried to one-up his boss by using the term 'Wuhan virus' only to be called out by China Foreign Ministry spokesman Geng Shuang who said it would 'stigmatise' his country.

'Despite the fact that the WHO has officially named this novel type of coronavirus, (a) certain American politician, disrespecting science and the WHO decision, jumped at the first chance to stigmatize China and Wuhan with it. We condemn this despicable practice,' said Shuang.

'No less (an) authority than the Chinese Communist Party said it came from Wuhan,' Pompeo told CNBC. 'So don't take Mike Pompeo's word for it. We have pretty high confidence that we know where this began.'

The sparring resulted in China walking back the idea that the outbreak even began in Wuhan. A tweet from China's official Twitter account on 4 March 2020, said it was 'still tracing the origin' of the virus, adding: 'Its origin is not necessarily in China.'

China's ambassador to South Africa tried the same reasoning, saying in a tweet: 'Although the epidemic first broke out in China, it did not necessarily mean that the virus is originated from China, let alone "made in China".'

Beijing was clearly trying to take the higher ground with another Foreign Ministry spokesperson Zhao Lijian saying at a press conference: 'The epidemic is a global challenge. The right move should be working together to fight it, which means no place for rumours and prejudice. We need science, reason and cooperation to drive out ignorance and bias.'

Trump refused to back down from the lab leak theory, even when the US national intelligence director's office said that while it was still investigating the origins of the virus it was certain it 'was not manmade or genetically modified'.

It is normal for presidents to stand by their spooks, but not Trump. At a White House press briefing at the end of April 2020, he was asked by a reporter: 'Have you seen anything at this point that gives you a high degree of confidence that the Wuhan Institute of Virology was the origin of this virus?'

'Yes, I have. Yes, I have,' Trump replied. 'And I think the World Health Organization should be ashamed of themselves because they're like the public relations agency for China ... Whether they (China) made a mistake, or whether it started off as a mistake and then they made another one, or did somebody do something on purpose?'

Asked to explain further, he said only: 'I can't tell you that. I'm not allowed to tell you that.'

This was manna from heaven for conspiracy theorists – a president hinting at a conspiracy without offering any details. It was an invitation for anyone with an agenda to fill in the gaps and it only fuelled the mainstream media's mistrust of a man who they felt played fast and loose with the truth.

What Trump had been privy to but couldn't say at the time was that the Pentagon's spy arm, the US Defense Intelligence Agency, had quietly updated its assessment of the cause of the pandemic to include the possibility that the virus could have been accidentally released from a lab in Wuhan.

The 27 March report titled 'China: Origins of COVID-19 Outbreak Remain Unknown', changed its original wording, according to *Newsweek*, from its assessment in January in which it 'judged that the outbreak probably occurred naturally' to concede it may have leaked 'accidentally' because of 'unsafe laboratory practices' in Wuhan.

The report claimed that American and Chinese scientists discovered that 'about 33 per cent of the original 41 identified cases did not have direct exposure' to the wet market, raising major question markets about the widely accepted 'wild' origin theory.

It added, however: 'We have no credible evidence to indicate SARS-CoV-2 was released intentionally or was created as a biological weapon. It is very unlikely that researchers or the Chinese government would intentionally release such a dangerous virus, especially within China, without possessing a known and effective vaccine.'

It would be another year before the lab theory was no longer regarded as a crackpot idea dreamed up by commie-hating conservatives, the media was suddenly looking at it more dispassionately and Joe Biden, now President Joe Biden, was ordering an official investigation by his intelligence chiefs into that self-same lab leak theory that he, like many others, had loudly condemned Trump for supporting.

What seems clear now is that Trump's flexible handle on the truth and his xenophobic language meant that by the time he spoke out to ask reasonable and well-founded questions about COVID's origins, he was scorned and ignored. Maybe that comes with the territory when you are playing the kind of divide and conquer political games that Trump appears to thrive on, but the result seems to be that there was a massive delay before the Chinese were facing the kind of pressure required for them to consider opening up their labs and scientific records and allowing the truth to be told. Only then could the world's scientists know they had all the known facts to try and fight the virus scourge.

And every additional day they were kept in the dark, thousands more innocent people were dying.

CHAPTER 9:

THE 'PATIENT ZERO' WHO NEVER GOT COVID
– 25 October 2019

After falling on the final lap in her bid for cycling gold in the 2019 Military World Games in Wuhan, US Army Sergeant 1st Class Maatje Benassi thought the worst was over when she bravely carried on to cross the finish line.

But as medics tended to her injuries, the Army reservist could never have known that her heroics on the track would trigger a chain of events that would leave her fearing for her life and put her at the centre of a major diplomatic row between the US and China over the origin of COVID-19.

To her colleagues on the American military cycling team – and everyone who knew her – Benassi was a tough competitor with a big heart and incredible stamina.

To the Chinese government, she was patient zero in the coronavirus pandemic.

Benassi led the pack of cyclists from around the world for most of the third and fourth laps of the five-lap, fifty-mile road race around Wuhan on 25 October 2019, and had just dropped back for a breather when disaster struck.

There were just two more wide turns on the road along part of Wuhan's East Lake to the finish just two kilometres away. 'My plan was to move up on the left,' Benassi told US Department of Defense News. 'And so if you move on the left, you don't have to hit your brakes; you can carry all that momentum – that speed – going into the turn.'

Just at that point, with Benassi poised to lead the US to gold, she said, 'It got really sketchy.' Going full speed into the right turn, a competitor in white came right up behind and hit her rear wheel, taking her down head-first. As she slammed into the ground, she heard a click 'and I knew I broke the helmet at that point'.

Her immediate fear was what other damage had she done as she struggled to breathe. 'I just had to catch my breath, but it wouldn't come,' she recalled. Despite being in terrible pain from bruised ribs, Benassi waved off colleagues who ran to her aid and wobbled to the finish in last place among the thirty competitors from eleven countries in the race.

'My goal was to finish it ... I came this far, I trained this hard, I had to finish it,' she told DoD News later. 'I was in a lot of pain, and my bike was rubbing, too ... Nothing went smooth, but I said, "Forget it, I'm just going to finish."'

The US team finished eighth in the race behind winners China and the non-commissioned officer from the 312th Observer-Controller-Trainer unit at Fort Meade, Maryland, returned home after a couple of days bruised and a little battered but otherwise none the worse for wear.

Somehow – certainly for no logical reason – Benassi had been singled out by George Webb, an online 'investigative journalist' who read the report about her cycling calamity and used it to spread a conspiracy theory linking her to an unsubstantiated claim that US military members in Wuhan for the games had brought the coronavirus to China.

Webb posted the claim on his YouTube video channel with 98,000 subscribers several months later in March 2020. 'Meet Wuhan Patient Zero Maatje Benassi,' he claimed in his now deleted post without any apparent evidence, linking her to a European DJ called Benny Benassi and saying both were part of the plot even though they are not related and did not know one another. Webb claimed Benny Benassi was the first Dutchman with coronavirus, but Benassi told CNN that one, he is Italian, and two, he hadn't had COVID. Asked by CNN what basis he had for accusing Maatje Benassi of carrying COVID to Wuhan, Webb insisted, 'There's a lot of circumstantial evidence and then there's a source here that I cannot reveal.' Although Benassi said she has never contracted the virus, Webb was adamant he had a 'source' at the Fort Belvoir Community Hospital in the US who told him she had tested positive. The claims, as absurd as they were, were picked up by the Chinese Communist Party media and YouTube videos featuring the baseless allegations were uploaded to social media platforms such as Weibo, WeChat and Xigua Video. Chillingly, comments about the posts included threats on Benassi's life.

'It's like waking up from a bad dream going into a nightmare day after day,' she told CNN in April 2020.

Her husband, Matt, tried his best to shut Webb down but kept hitting obstacles as the YouTuber kept doubling down on his allegations. 'We are interwoven into his storyline now,' Matt told CNN. 'He is never going to give it up.'

The Chinese, desperate to divert attention away from their

own role in the coronavirus crisis, latched on to the fact that Benassi and other US competitors in Wuhan worked near to Fort Detrick in Maryland, the headquarters of a military germ lab about fifty miles outside Washington with a spotty safety history. In August 2019, the United States Army Medical Research Institute in Fort Detrick shut down research over safety concerns.

The Centers for Disease Control and Prevention ordered the temporary closure at the lab – which experimented on potentially deadly organisms such as the Ebola virus, smallpox and anthrax – because its labs didn't have 'sufficient systems in place to decontaminate wastewater'.

The lab insisted there had been no leaks and no risks to public health, but it provided a circumstantial opportunity for the Chinese to launch a propaganda counter-offensive against Trump and his claims of a 'Kung-Flu' virus by suggesting the American team at the military games may have been infected.

China's claims on social media became increasingly bizarre, including a tweet by Department of Information Counsellor Li Yang trying to suggest the pandemic's origins had something to do with people in Wisconsin suffering from EVALI, a lung disease associated with vaping.

The tweet read: 'The whole world needs the answer: e-cigarettes are sold all over the world. Why are there a large number of e-cigarette pneumonia cases only near Fort Detrick in the US? What's the relationship between Fort Detrick and the coronavirus pandemic?'

The answer would be that the quoted e-cigarette pneumonia cases 'only near Fort Detrick' were in fact nearly 1,000 miles away. So probably no relationship then!

A Russian YouTube channel also claimed there was a

COVID-19 outbreak at a care home near Fort Detrick without any evidence.

As crazy as some of the claims were, the Fort Detrick theory initially caught fire in March 2020 when China's Foreign Ministry spokesperson Zhao Lijian tweeted an article blaming the US base to his nearly one million followers.

China's ambassador to the US Cui Tiankai told *Axios on HBO* that he believed it was 'crazy' to spread rumours that the virus originated in America but as the Trump administration increasingly turned its venom on China, the Chinese media machine appeared to pick up the Fort Detrick line and run with it.

According to Bret Schafer, a media and disinformation fellow at the Alliance for Securing Democracy, at least thirty-five key Chinese officials and state media outlets mentioned Fort Detrick in more than 115 tweets in nine languages after a later Zhao press conference in May 2021 when he sought to rev up the speculation, saying: 'What secrets are hidden in the suspicion-shrouded Fort Detrick and the over 200 US bio-labs all over the world?' Writing in *Foreign Policy*, Schafer said that in a year-long campaign beginning in March 2020, more than 400 articles, videos, tweets and press conferences involving Chinese government officials and state-linked media mentioned Fort Detrick. They include the conspiracy theory that Maatje Benassi brought the virus to Wuhan from the Fort Detrick area. 'Whether or not these efforts are coordinated at the state level is unclear,' wrote Schafer. 'However, numerous studies, including one I co-wrote, have highlighted Beijing's willingness to manufacture consensus through the use of coordinated inauthentic behaviour. In the case of Fort Detrick narratives, there are several examples of Chinese officials retweeting suspicious accounts. 'It's easy to poke holes in Beijing's Fort Detrick narratives,' he continued, 'starting with the fact that the two labs studying coronaviruses in the United States are in Galveston, Texas, and Chapel Hill, North Carolina – not Frederick, Maryland.

'But with influence operations, soundness of logic is less important than repetition. Beijing's efforts to carpet bomb information platforms with theories – however implausible – about Fort Detrick's role in the global pandemic have borne some fruit. In January, after Hua Chunying, another spokesperson for the Chinese Ministry of Foreign Affairs, repeated false claims about Fort Detrick, the lab topped the trending topic chart on Weibo, a major Chinese social media platform.

'And the effect is not limited to China. According to Google Trends, the topic and query terms most associated with Google searches for "Fort Detrick" over the past two years were "Wuhan" and "coronavirus" respectively.'

Marcel Schliebs, a researcher at the University of Oxford, uncovered a network of over 550 pro-China Twitter accounts that spread a nearly identical message with disinformation about the coronavirus translated into a number of different languages at the same times every day. 'Attribution is really difficult,' Schliebs, a postdoctoral researcher of computational propaganda at Oxford's Programme on Democracy and Technology, told NBC News. 'But we can see there's a coordinated effort, and that it's a pro-Chinese narrative.'

One of the most bizarre theories that Schliebs discovered was tweeted by Zha Liyou, the Chinese Consul General in Kolkata in India, claiming that a shipment of Maine lobsters sent to Wuhan in November 2019 was the cause of the outbreak. The unsubstantiated accusation stems in part from a World Health

Organization report that there is a 'scientific basis for the possibility' that seafood imports could transmit coronavirus because SARS-CoV-2 can survive for long periods in frozen and refrigerated products. A spokesperson for the Maine Center for Disease Control had an icy response to the rumours. 'It's a right load of codswallop,' he said.

The general assumption when we discuss conspiracy theories is that they are conjured up by disenfranchised individuals unhappy or even enraged at the governments they see as hiding the truth from them. Here, it seems certain that the Chinese, one of the most powerful nations on earth, was involved in a systematic attempt to mislead the world by spinning a conspiracy theory they knew was patently false. As we will see, they were far from alone among governments spreading false stories for their own ends.

At the same time, we also had Donald Trump in the White House spreading any number of falsehoods, including early boasts that the pandemic was under control and equivalent to the flu, democracy-challenging claims of a 'stolen' election and even bonkers ideas like the noise from windmills causing cancer.

These are government-sponsored conspiracy theories. They aren't honest challenges to an accepted narrative. They certainly aren't determined attempts, whether justified or ill-advised, to get to the truth or to right a wrong.

There's nothing new here. Leaders have been fibbing to us since the beginning of time, but social media has given them the means of reaching millions of people around the globe with the concept that if enough mud is flung far and often enough some of it is bound to stick. Ironically, one of the chief tools that the Chinese used to spread their misinformation about Fort Detrick and other COVID theories was Twitter, the platform its own ordinary citizens have been banned from using since 2009.

So, if we can't believe the leaders of superpowers like China and the United States, who can we believe?

Don't get me started on Russia and Vladimir Putin.

Or Boris Johnson.

CHAPTER 10:

RIDDLE ME THIS, WHEN IS A CONSPIRACY THEORY NOT A CONSPIRACY THEORY?

– 23 May 2021

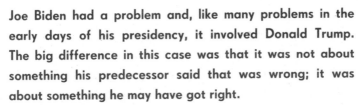

Joe Biden had a problem and, like many problems in the early days of his presidency, it involved Donald Trump. The big difference in this case was that it was not about something his predecessor said that was wrong; it was about something he may have got right.

Biden was well aware of a State Department fact sheet that was circulated towards the end of the Trump presidency suggesting that several researchers at the Wuhan Institute of Virology where 'Bat Woman' Shi Zhengli and her team had been working on the bat samples from the Tongguan mine had fallen sick in the autumn of 2019. Details were vague, but the intelligence report said the lab staff were ill 'with symptoms consistent with both COVID-19 and common seasonal illness'.

Even though Trump had been unusually reticent in revealing his source, the fact sheet had been the basis for his claims and those of his close confidants like Senator Tom Cotton that a lab leak could have been the cause of the pandemic. The problem was that the kind of toxic language Trump used to make his point led to claims of racism.

China's strong denials and the mainstream media's collective suspicions towards Trump had combined to relegate the idea to a conspiracy theory and, despite growing misgivings over the Wuhan wet market as the origin, its alternative was considered a political hot potato in the early days of the Biden administration. By giving the lab leak theory credibility, it was effectively conferring a propaganda triumph on Trump. It would even be seen by some Democrats as rubber-stamping Trump's xenophobia.

The truth was that America's intelligence services were split between the two theories and the intransigence by the Chinese who refused to make Shi or the lab records available to investigators meant they were stuck.

But on 23 May 2021, an exclusive report appeared in the *Wall Street Journal* that left Biden with little choice but to act. It said that three researchers from the Wuhan Institute had not only fallen sick in November 2019, but they were sick enough to need hospital treatment.

November was particularly significant because it fits in with the time period experts generally reckoned the SARS-CoV-2 virus first began circulating in Wuhan ahead of the first confirmed case on 8 December 2019.

The Chinese, adamant there was no leak from any of its laboratories, were quick to point to a report by the WHO following a visit to the Institute in February dismissing the idea that the pandemic emanated from its labs. Shi had told the WHO investigators that all her staff had tested negative for COVID-19 antibodies, a possible contradiction of the State Department fact sheet claim.

The WHO team had apparently believed the explanation they were given that the only illnesses suffered by researchers were the usual seasonal ailments and there was nothing connected to their SARS work. They concluded that a lab leak was 'extremely unlikely'.

But David Asher, who worked under Trump acolyte Mike Pompeo in the State Department and led a task force on the origins of the virus, said the researchers who fell ill could represent 'the first known cluster' of COVID-19 infections.

'I'm very doubtful that three people in highly protected circumstances in a level three laboratory working on coronaviruses would all get sick with influenza that put them in the hospital or in severe conditions all in the same week, and it didn't have anything to do with the coronavirus,' he told a Hudson Institute seminar, according to the *Wall Street Journal*.

The State Department fact sheet, it emerged, said the fact that researchers had been ill 'raises questions about the credibility' of Shi. The *Journal* said the Intelligence report also criticised China for its 'deceit and disinformation'.

The *WSJ* article jump-started the stalled lab leak theory and suddenly all the big news outlets were re-examining it and asking why it had been dismissed by so many for so long. The possibility of a lab leak was back at the top of the Washington news cycle and Joe Biden was being asked what he was going to do about it and why he wasn't putting enough pressure on Beijing to be more transparent.

'Wouldn't there naturally be quite a curiosity within the Biden administration that this could have come from a lab?' *Washington Post* reporter Annie Linskey asked White House

Press Secretary Jen Psaki. 'Nearly 600,000 people have died, and the president has shown an enormous amount of empathy for that. But should this be the cause, it would seem that the United States would want to put some of his intelligence firepower on to that question,' she added.

Psaki played a straight bat, shifting the blame to the WHO. 'We need access to the underlying data,' she answered. 'We need access to the information that the Chinese government has in order to make a determination through the international bodies that would do this investigation. And that's something we've called for many, many times. We've pressed with our international partners for the WHO to support an expert-driven evaluation of the pandemic's origins. We would certainly participate in that with all of our research resources from the United States.'

The previous day, Psaki had said the US had 'no means' to confirm that the lab workers mentioned in the *Journal* article got sick.

Dr Anthony Fauci, Biden's top adviser on the pandemic, had already made it public that he was 'not convinced' that the virus emerged naturally, adding, 'I think we should continue to investigate what went on in China until we find out to the best of our ability what happened.'

Fauci, the director of the US National Institute of Allergies and Infectious Diseases, added: 'Certainly, the people who investigated it say it likely was the emergence from an animal reservoir that then infected individuals, but it could have been something else, and we need to find that out. So, you know, that's the reason why I said I'm perfectly in favour of any investigation that looks into the origin of the virus.'

He was also pressed on the lab leak theory during an 11 May

2021 Senate hearing. 'Do you think it's possible that COVID-19 arose from a lab accident ... in Wuhan, and should it be fully investigated?' Senator Roger Marshall, a doctor, asked Fauci.

'That possibility certainly exists, and I am totally in favour of a full investigation of whether that could have happened,' replied Fauci, who had claimed earlier in the pandemic that he thought it more likely that COVID-19 'evolved in nature and then jumped species', and wasn't 'artificially or deliberately manipulated'.

The narrative was changing fast. On 26 May 2021 – three days after the *Journal* report was published – Biden decided he could no longer ignore the demands for action and gave his intelligence chiefs ninety days to report back to him on the relative merits of the two theories. While conceding the intelligence community 'coalesced around two likely scenarios' he took a veiled jab at Trump, saying: 'The failure to get our inspectors on the ground in those early months will always hamper any investigation into the origin of COVID-19.' US Health and Human Services Secretary Xavier Becerra also urged the WHO to go back and take a second look at the origins of the pandemic, saying: 'Phase 2 of the COVID origins study must be launched with terms of reference that are transparent, science-based and give international experts the independence to fully assess the source of the virus and the early days of the outbreak.' Unsurprisingly, Trump was quick to claim credit. 'Now everybody is agreeing that I was right when I very early on called Wuhan as the source of COVID-19, sometimes referred to as the China Virus,' he said in a statement. 'To me it was obvious from the beginning, but I was badly criticized, as usual. Now they are all saying, "He was right."'

Of course, nobody seriously questioned whether the pandemic started in Wuhan and Biden's intelligence review could never pin the origin on a lab leak but it did leave the theory on the table, officially elevating it from a conspiracy theory to a legitimate one.

In the 'declassified key takeaways' from the intelligence report, most agencies agreed with 'low confidence' that the Chinese didn't genetically engineer the virus and they were unanimous in believing it wasn't developed as a bioweapon.

Five intelligence agencies, including the national Intelligence Council, favoured the wild origin theory, according to the summary, but one US intelligence agency, which was not identified, assessed 'with moderate confidence that the first human infection with SARS-CoV-2 most likely was the result of a laboratory-associated incident, probably involving experimentation, animal handling, or sampling by the Wuhan Institute of Virology'. Crucially, all of the eighteen US intelligence agencies believed both theories to be plausible, but the summary accepted that they may never learn what really happened 'unless new information allows them to determine the specific pathway for initial natural contact with an animal or to determine that a laboratory in Wuhan was handling SARS-CoV-2 or a close progenitor virus before COVID-19 emerged'. While the lab leak theory may have officially come back into the reckoning, much of the scientific community was still convinced the wet market was to blame. Two extensive studies were released on 26 February 2022 that concluded that live animals sold in Wuhan were probably carrying the coronavirus.

The claim was based on the mapping of 156 cases of COVID reported in Wuhan in December 2019. By checking their latitude and longitude, researchers surmised the highest density of cases was around the market. Tracking another 736 cases in Wuhan in the following January and February showed the infections spreading out into areas of the city with high numbers of elderly residents.

The researchers also claimed that evidence from genetic samples showed that south-west areas of the market where racoon dogs and other wild animals were being sold in late 2019 showed traces of SARS-CoV-2. 'When you look at all of the evidence together, it's an extraordinarily clear picture that the pandemic started at the Huanan market,' Michael Worobey, an evolutionary biologist at the University of Arizona and a co-author of the studies, told the *New York Times*.

However, the reports were not published in a scientific journal and consequently were not peer reviewed. Any live animals that may have been at the market were also cleared out before investigators arrived to check into the possibility that it was the source of origin.

The debate will undoubtedly continue, based on the limited knowledge available without China's cooperation. Scientists – and anyone with common sense – will tell you that it is crucial to understand how the COVID-19 pandemic began so we can do everything possible to ensure it never happens again.

But it is very likely that the only people who do know what happened have been sworn to silence in China. And the rest of us have little choice but to keep guessing ...

CHAPTER 11:

CAN YOU HEAR ME NOW?
– 4 April 2020

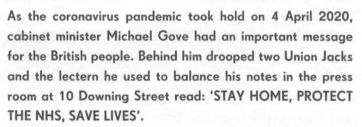

As the coronavirus pandemic took hold on 4 April 2020, cabinet minister Michael Gove had an important message for the British people. Behind him drooped two Union Jacks and the lectern he used to balance his notes in the press room at 10 Downing Street read: 'STAY HOME, PROTECT THE NHS, SAVE LIVES'.

With a live television audience waiting with bated breath, Gove wasted no time. He was determined to put down a conspiracy theory linking the spread of coronavirus with 5G phone technology that had caused a series of violent incidents across the country.

Mobile phone masks had been attacked and people were demanding action from the government. Gove called the theory 'dangerous nonsense' and handed the mic over to Professor Stephen Powis, the national medical director of the National Health Service, to, as the Cabinet Minister put it, 'say a little bit more about the vital importance of knocking down this rubbish'.

'So, the 5G story is complete and utter rubbish,' started Powis. 'It's nonsense. It's the worst kind of fake news. The reality is that the mobile phone networks are absolutely critical to all of us, particularly at a time when we are asking people to stay at home and to not see relatives and friends. But, in particular, those are the phone networks that are used by our emergency services and our health workers. I'm absolutely outraged, absolutely disgusted, that people would be taking action against the very infrastructure that we need to respond to this health emergency.'

It had come to something when the government used prime-time TV in the middle of a crisis to try and counteract what appeared on the surface to be a conspiracy theory born of paranoia. But the idea that 5G was behind the pandemic's inexorable spread had moved beyond the armchair troublemakers on the internet and into action. Three recent mobile phone mast fires were being treated by police as arson, the most recent blaze in Spencer's Lane in Aintree, Liverpool, close to the M57 motorway.

Nor were the rumours that 5G was causing coronavirus symptoms restricted to anonymous names on social media. Singer Keri Hilson tweeted to her 4.2 million followers on 15 March 2020, that, 'People have been trying to warn us about 5G for YEARS. Petitions, organizations, studies ... what we're going thru is the affects [sic] of radiation. 5G launched in CHINA. Nov 1, 2019. People dropped dead. See attached & go to my IG stories for more. TURN OFF 5G by disabling LTE!!!'

Popular rapper Wiz Khalifa tweeted on 3 April 2020: 'Corona? 5g? Or both?'

After a mast was set ablaze in Belfast, voices were caught on tape shouting 'Fuck the 5G' and 'Viva la revolution'.

Days later, a third twenty-metre (seventy-foot) mast that was serving Birmingham's Nightingale Hospital, built to treat coronavirus patients, was attacked by arsonists. In a 14 April LinkedIn post, Vodafone UK's chief executive Nick Jeffery wrote that it was 'heart-rending enough that families cannot be there at the bedside of loved ones who are critically ill. It's even more upsetting that even the small solace of a phone or video call may now be denied them because of the selfish actions of a few deluded conspiracy theorists.'

He added: 'Burning down masts means damaging important national infrastructure. In practice, this means families not being able to say a final goodbye to their loved ones; hard-working doctors, nurses and police officers not being able to phone their kids, partners or parents for a comforting chat. Arsonists, please think about what you are doing and stop.'

Telecoms engineers complained they were being abused in the streets by people saying they were causing the coronavirus. Many of the razed towers weren't even 5G but the more traditional 3G and 4G service. One video, watched over 2.5 million times, shows a woman telling telecom workers they're going to 'kill everyone'. The unseen woman approaches two men laying cable in an urban street during a lockdown. 'Do you work for the NHS?' she asks and when the men tell her they are laying 5G optic cables, she continues, 'But you're not supposed to be within two metres of each other. Is this essential work?

'You know that you are laying 5G?' she continues. 'You know that kills people? You know when they turn this on it's going to kill everyone? That's why they are building the hospitals.

'How do you feel? Do you have children? Do you have parents? How do you feel that when they turn that switch on, bye, bye, Mama? Are you content to continue doing that job? Are they paying you well enough to kill her?

'You have just admitted that you are laying 5G so that's basically why we are all inside while you have free rein of London.'

'Everyone wants 5G,' says the bemused worker.

'Well, everyone will be dead,' continues the woman, 'So who's going to be playing on the internet, who's going to be on their PlayStations? We'll all be in hospital on breathing apparatus. Why do you think they are building 25,000 sort of concentration camps of death in the London ExCeL right now? It's because of this wire here.

'I'm not having a go at you guys. I'm just saying that it's honestly just what you're doing. It's dangerous. I'm glad that you've told me what you're doing but, ultimately, it's a disgrace.'

Writing in the *Mail on Sunday* in early April 2020, BT chief executive Philip Jansen said that thirty-nine of his company engineers had been verbally or physically assaulted, including some who faced death threats, by anti-5G protesters and eleven BT mobile masts had been destroyed or damaged through arson. 'The most bizarre theory, and one that brought a rare smile in these dark times, was that the wonderful tradition we've so quickly established of clapping at 8pm on a Thursday to show our appreciation for the NHS and other key workers, is actually done to create enough noise to mask the "loud beeping" of 5G networks being tested,' he wrote.

'We all need to be able to recognise conspiracy theories, and to stop them before they become harmful,' he concluded. 'They are just like a virus – if we starve them of the ability to reach new people, they will die out, and we can all focus on coming together as one nation to get through these most challenging of times.'

The issue was that there was no absolute science proving

that 5G was harmless, even if it didn't cause COVID. It's a new technology and enough time hasn't passed for its effects to be fully examined. TV presenter Eamonn Holmes, about as reliable a figure as you will find in British broadcasting, appeared to be sharing similar sentiments to that in a controversial exchange with consumer editor Alice Beer on his *This Morning* daytime show on 13 April 2020.

Former BBC *Watchdog* presenter Beer maintained the theory that 5G caused coronavirus was 'not true and incredibly stupid'.

Holmes, perhaps voicing the thoughts of many viewers, told his colleague: 'I totally agree with everything you are saying. But what I don't accept is mainstream media immediately slapping that down as not true when they don't know it's not true. No one should attack or damage or do anything like that, but it's very easy to say it is not true because it suits the state narrative.'

The backlash to his remarks was so strong that Holmes returned to the topic on the following day's show to say he had been 'misinterpreted'.

'For the avoidance of any doubt, I want to make it completely clear there's no scientific evidence to substantiate any of those 5G theories,' he added. That didn't stop him and his ITV bosses getting a rap on the knuckles from the broadcasting watchdog Ofcom, which said: 'In our view, Eamonn Holmes' ambiguous comments were ill-judged and risked undermining viewers' trust in advice from public authorities and scientific evidence. His statements were also highly sensitive in view of the recent attacks on mobile phone masts in the UK, caused by conspiracy theories linking 5G technology and the virus.

'Broadcasters have editorial freedom to discuss and challenge the approach taken by public authorities to a serious public health crisis such as the coronavirus. However, discussions about unproven claims and theories which could undermine viewers' trust in official public health information must be put fully into context to ensure viewers are protected.'

As emphatic as the British government and telecom bosses were about the 'rubbish' 5G theory, concern about the effects of mobile phones and sound waves are hardly new. I worked for a Fleet Street editor in the 1990s who commissioned stories on a weekly basis about the possible dangers to conception by carrying a mobile in your pocket, about the jeopardy your brain was in by putting your phone to the ear, about the cancers you risked by straying from the landline. None of the claims had much scientific basis as it was in the early days of the technology, but the editor was relentless. He was convinced that science had just not caught up to the dangers and that by the time it did it could be too late.

Twenty years before the pandemic, Broward County schools district in Florida was warned not to offer laptops and wireless networks in its classrooms because the technology represented 'a serious health hazard' to its 250,000 students. Physicist Bill Curry claimed the risk of radiation affecting the brain grew with the strength of the wireless reception. Radio waves could result in brain cancer, he argued. A chart in his report, captioned, 'Microwave Absorption in Brain Tissue', claimed to show a rise in the damage to brain tissue corresponding to the rising frequency of radio waves. 'This graph shows why I am concerned,' Curry wrote. He warned that children were especially vulnerable, adding: 'Their brains are developing.'

Curry's findings were amplified by alarmists and used to bolster arguments against wireless technology. In 2011, they were used to support a lawsuit seeking to force public schools in Portland, Oregon, to shut down its wireless network. They became so well known they were accepted as fact in many scientific circles even though other experts had been sceptical over his methodology.

Harvard-educated scientist Dr David O. Carpenter took up the cause, writing in 2013: 'The rapid increase in the use of cell phones increases risk of cancer, male infertility, and neurobehavioral abnormalities.'

With the growth of 4G and then 5G, Russian media began running stories warning of the threat from wireless technology. 'The higher the frequency, the more dangerous it is to living organisms,' claimed a segment on the Russian news channel RT. US intelligence sources say Russia's attempts to sabotage America's confidence in 5G came from the very top and was part of Vladimir Putin's campaign to destabilise his superpower rivals in Washington. Russia is way behind in its 5G roll-out and is purposeful in its attempts to discredit and undermine its growth in the West. Molly McKew, head of Fianna Strategies, a US consulting firm that seeks to counter Russian disinformation, told the *New York Times* that the Kremlin 'would really enjoy getting democratic governments tied up in fights over 5G's environmental and health hazards'.

5G is the fifth generation of mobile phone technology so the science has had plenty of time to catch up, but its critics would still argue that it's a multi-billion-pound industry and that darker motives were behind the dearth of publicly available research. Yes, they provide exponentially faster downloads and uploads but at what price, they argued?

In March 2018, the story my old editor had been waiting for finally came around. A scientific peer review gave credibility to a US government study that concluded there was 'clear evidence' that radiation from mobile phones causes cancer. Eleven independent scientists spent three days investigating the study by the US Department of Health and Social Services' National Toxicology Program. The largest ever experiment of its kind basically exposed mice to levels of radiation they estimated to be equal to an average mobile phone user's lifetime exposure.

The resulting heart tissue cancer they found in those rats, they insisted, was way higher than any random occurrence could explain. The scientists also found some evidence of cancer in the brain and adrenal glands, according to a report in *The Observer*. The authors of the article, Mark Hertsgaard, environment correspondent for the Nation, and author and 'investigative historian' Mark Dowie, argued that the wireless industry had used big tobacco techniques through the years to hide the true effects of wireless from an unsuspecting public, writing: 'Lack of definitive proof that a technology is harmful does not mean the technology is safe, yet the wireless industry has succeeded in selling this logical fallacy to the world.

'The upshot is that, over the past thirty years, billions of people around the world have been subjected to a public health experiment: use a mobile phone today, find out later if it causes genetic damage or cancer. Meanwhile, the industry has obstructed a full understanding of the science and news organisations have failed to inform the public about what scientists really think.'

A week after the report appeared in the *Observer*, its editors clearly felt the need to run a follow-up story carrying the opposing argument. Dr David Robert Grimes, a physicist, cancer researcher and science writer based at Queen's University Belfast and the University of Oxford, accused the authors of 'scaremongering', and claimed the previous week's report was 'strewn with rudimentary errors and dubious inferences'.

Grimes acknowledged the public's health concerns, saying of

the article about the study: 'Its powerful narrative tapped into rich themes; our deep-seated fears about cancer, corporate greed and technology's potentially noxious influence on our health. It spread rapidly across social media – facilitated by the very object on which it cast doubt.'

But he continued: 'The opening paragraph lays bare a seemingly astounding conclusion – the US's National Toxicology Program concluded that mobile phones cause cancer. This is, to put it charitably, a devious extrapolation. The study in question observed that rats exposed to intense radiofrequency (RF) had slightly higher rates of brain cancers relative to the control group. But far from being a smoking gun, the flaws in this study paint a muddled picture. First, the preprint reveals that the rats in the RF-exposure group lived significantly longer than those controls. As cancer is primarily correlated with age, it's not surprising the longer-lived group would get more cancer, but it would be equally daft to presume RF increases lifespan based on these results.'

He also pointed to a Danish study that followed 358,403 people for twenty-seven years and found no link between cancer and mobile phones.

Published on 21 July 2018, Grimes' concluding paragraph is remarkably prescient. 'Scaremongering narratives may be more alluring than the less sensational, scientific findings, but they are not harmless,' he wrote. 'We need only look at any vaccine panic to see the cost in human life when superstition outpaces science. In an age where misinformation can perpetuate rapidly, it can be difficult to parse fact from fiction, but it's imperative that we hone our scientific scepticism rather than succumb to baseless panics – our very wellbeing depends on it.'

Less than two years later, Michael Gove would be on television trying to make that same argument that there was no evidence that wireless technology was unsafe. And conspiracy theorists would still be quoting that twenty-year-old graph by Bill Curry saying that the higher the radio wave frequency the higher the risk of cancer. It was one of the most quoted theories backing the idea that super-high frequency 5G was to blame for the spread of the coronavirus.

It didn't seem to matter that Dr Curry's graph had been discredited in some quarters. In a July 2019 article in the *New York Times*, experts on the biological effects of electromagnetic radiation insisted radio waves became less dangerous the higher the frequency, as long as they are not extreme high frequencies such as X-rays. Curry's report, said the experts, didn't consider the protective value of the human skin and its 'shielding effect' from radiation. 'In time, echoes of his reports fed Russian news sites noted for stoking misinformation about 5G technology,' said *The Times*. 'What began as a simple graph became a case study in how bad science can take root and flourish.'

Again, this was published months before the first victims were admitted to hospital in Wuhan with symptoms that would become synonymous with COVID.

COVID provided especially fertile ground for the conspiracy theorists. As with most theories lacking any substantiated proof, they ranged from the bonkers – the virus is a bioweapon being spread via the mobile masts to thin out the world's population – to the theoretically possible, such as suggesting a link between 5G waves and its effect on the body's immune system. Proponents of this theory point to maps of the United States that show the areas that were worst hit by COVID also had the highest 5G coverage. Of course, that premise falls down because the bigger cities and towns are more likely to have 5G and those same densely populated areas would naturally be hit hardest by the pandemic. The outbreak also soon spread to countries such as Iran and India where 5G coverage was negligible at the time.

Many people who were convinced that 5G was to blame for the pandemic quoted controversial French virologist Luc Montagnier, winner of the Nobel Prize in 2008 for the discovery of HIV, who claimed that bacteria could generate radio waves. His view, by no means accepted by many mainstream biologists, was that some bacterial DNA continued to send electromagnetic signals even after an infection had cleared up.

The late Nobel laureate, who died in a suburb of Paris in February 2022, moved to Jiaotong University in Shanghai after his funding dried up in his home country and refused to back down on his more sensational claims, saying: 'I'm a gambler out for the big killing. Like a roulette player at the table, I'm addicted to getting results out of my laboratory.'

The French may also have first directed suspicion at the 5G mobile masts. A conspiracy website called Les Moutons Enragés – 'The Rabid Sheep' – posted on 20 January 2020 that 5G towers were built in Wuhan soon before the first coronavirus cases. Two days later, a Belgian newspaper ran an interview with a physician linking the Wuhan 5G masts with the outbreak. Although the article was quickly taken down, it wasn't in time to prevent social media from spreading it to conspiracy theorists worldwide. Among Facebook groups set up to protest 5G were 'Stop 5G Global Community' with over 8,000 members and 'Lawful Stop5G Rebellion No Violence' with over 35,000 followers, 'Stop 5G International', 'Global Action to Stop 5G' and 'Anti-Wireless Shop'.

The 'Stop 5G Group' with about 60,000 members, and

'Destroy 5G Save Our Children' were among the organisations that were later targeted and removed by Facebook after they were found to be carrying comments encouraging the vandalism of wireless masts.

According to data collected between 1 January and 20 April 2020, by Zignal Labs and published by Recode, the idea that 5G causes COVID-19 was the second most popular conspiracy theory with 1,062,192 mentions (the most popular, with 1,382,889 mentions was the theory that Bill Gates created the virus).

The counter-offensive on the 5G conspiracy didn't appear to have done much good. In the days after Gove's press conference, another seventeen 5G masts were damaged or destroyed and, to date, there have been more than eighty-seven arson attacks on mobile phone towers in the UK alone. The great irony is that the reason the 5G rumours spread so quickly and so effectively was because of the speed of the internet network. And when the mobile masts burned, who was the first to complain that their phones weren't working? The modern conspiracy theorist, after all, is a creature of social media and theories about 5G continue to get a good reception even now.

CHAPTER 12:

DONALD TRUMP, KING OF THE CONSPIRACY THEORISTS
– 2 October 2020

▼

Donald Trump's extraordinary rise to power began with his baseless claim that Barack Obama was not a US citizen and resulted in him questioning the election results in the world's defining democracy. But he has also fuelled endless conspiracy theories about COVID-19, pointing a finger of suspicion at the Chinese for starting the pandemic, pushing hydroxychloroquine and bleach as a cure, and generally downplaying the threat even as the numbers of deaths and infections piled up across the world.

The theories reached their zenith on 2 October 2020, after it was confirmed that Trump and First Lady Melania had contracted the virus. He had spent much of the year trying to play down the virus as little more than overblown flu and claiming credit for shutting down America's borders way after that particular horse had bolted. Now his supporters were hailing him a genius for catching COVID, claiming it was a) part of a cunning plot to show the world how easy it could be 'cured' or b) part of a Machiavellian plan to infect Joe Biden during a late September televised head-to-head presidential debate and kill off his older rival for the White House.

The conspiracy theories weren't restricted to the right or left, but the hashtag #TrumpCOVIDHoax' was trending on Twitter in the US all that day. On his Facebook page, according to VOX, left-wing *Fahrenheit 11/9* filmmaker Michael Moore said he couldn't even trust Trump to tell the truth about being sick and feared he was just using it to divert attention away from a dip in the polls. 'There is one absolute truth about Trump,' he wrote. 'He is a consistent, absolute, unrelenting, fearless, and professional liar ... Trump has a history of lying about his health ... He may have it. But it's also possible he's lying. That's just a fact.'

Moore continued: 'HE MAY USE THIS TO PUSH FOR DELAYING/POSTPONING THE ELECTION. The constitution does not allow for this, but he doesn't give a f*ck about the constitution. He and his thug Attorney General [William] Barr have no shame and will stop at nothing to stay in power.'

Bette Midler, the left-leaning actress and singer, tweeted to her two million followers: 'Timing's so interesting. I guess Trump's quarantining will mean no rallies, and no more debates. Convenient.'

Right-wingers insisted Trump had been targeted as part of an elaborate plot to sabotage his presidential campaign and guarantee a Biden victory, forgetting that the president had been largely ignoring the precautionary advice of his own medical staff since the pandemic took hold.

Conservative commentator and former GOP congressional candidate DeAnna Lorraine had no doubt that Trump had COVID, but she suggested China was to blame for trying to bump off the president. She also seemed to think that only Republicans had caught it.

'Could Trump catching COVID-19 technically be viewed as an assassination attempt on our President by the Chinese?' Lorraine tweeted, adding: 'Does anyone else find it odd that no prominent Democrats have had the virus, but the list of Republicans goes on and on?'

If it wasn't the Chinese, Lorraine suggested the left were also in the frame. The rumour doing the rounds was that a COVID-tainted 'rag' was used to wipe down the podium and mic that Trump used in his presidential debate in Cleveland, Ohio, on 29 September 2020.

'I'm just going to say what we're all thinking,' she posted after hearing Trump had tested positive. 'Trump was fine until the debate, where they set up microphones and podiums for him. Incubation period is usually two to three days. He tests positive a couple of days after the debate. I put nothing past the left. NOTHING.'

Late-night comedian Jimmy Kimmel had his own take on her tweets, saying: 'Well, I wouldn't say we were all thinking that, might just be you. You know what else is odd. It's odd when skydivers who use parachutes come down fine but the ones who don't get splattered like a bag of coleslaw.'

Bear in mind, by the way, this woman had more than 400,000 followers. So, she wasn't tweeting in a vacuum.

Trump didn't need supporters or foes to make up conspiracy theories about him; he was quite adept at inventing his own. On 31 October 2020, he told a campaign rally in Michigan that doctors were diagnosing cases of COVID because it paid them more. 'Our doctors get more money if someone dies from COVID,' he said, giving national attention to a fringe conspiracy theory that few people had taken seriously previously. The American Medical Association was quick to strike back at Trump, tweeting: 'Rather than attacking and lobbing baseless charges at physicians, our leaders should be following the science.'

Joe Biden, in the final days of a tight White House race with Trump, went straight on the offensive, saying: 'The President of the United States is accusing the medical profession of making up COVID deaths so they make more money. Doctors and nurses go to work every day to save lives. They do their jobs. Donald Trump should stop attacking them and do his job.'

But Trump was clearly looking at COVID to get voters back onside. His poll numbers were falling and his personal attacks on 'Sleepy Joe' Biden, while effective to a degree, had not fatally wounded an opponent at the wrong end of his seventies. Trump settled on a strategy to politicise the pandemic. It would have some serious consequences in Washington, D.C. as Republicans increasingly lined up with Trump against COVID precautions such as masks and vaccinations while Democrats took a more cautionary approach. At the heart of almost every COVID clash, it seemed, was another conspiracy theory.

'We have made tremendous progress with the China Virus, but the Fake News refuses to talk about it this close to the Election,' Trump tweeted on 26 October 2020, adding: 'COVID, COVID, COVID is being used by them, in total coordination, in order to change our great early election numbers. Should be an election law violation!'

Trump argued that the only reason the infection numbers were rising to record highs was because America was doing more tests, an easily proved fallacy. 'Cases up because we TEST, TEST, TEST. A Fake News Media Conspiracy,' Trump tweeted. 'Many young people who heal very fast. 99.9 per cent. Corrupt

Media conspiracy at all time high. On November 4th., topic will totally change. VOTE!'

Days later, he claimed: 'You know why we have so many case numbers? Because we do more testing than any country in the world ... there's plenty good about testing, too. The bad thing is you find cases.'

Experts were quick to point out that the spike in cases was way greater than the number of tests, but the experts weren't Trump's target audience. He couldn't care less what they said – his supporters were eating it up. At a campaign rally in Allentown, Pennsylvania, attendees told BuzzFeed that the virus was infringing on their freedoms. 'It's 24/7 and I think it's used to keep everybody scared to death, scared to walk out of their house. I think they're using it to control us. Everybody's scared to death to live their lives the way they used to,' said David Mitchell, fifty-eight, from New Jersey.

Trump, as always, the conspiracy theorists dream, taunted controversial cures from the Oval Office. Long before he tested positive, Trump suggested in April 2020 that injecting disinfectant as a treatment might be a good idea. It came during a White House coronavirus task force briefing when officials discussed government research showing the virus may weaken under heat and sunlight. The study also showed bleach and isopropyl alcohol could kill the virus in saliva.

'So, supposing we hit the body with a tremendous – whether it's ultraviolet or just very powerful light,' said the president. Turning to White House coronavirus response coordinator Dr Deborah Birx, he continued: 'And I think you said that hasn't been checked but you're going to test it? And then I said, supposing you brought the light inside of the body, which you can do either through the skin or in some other way. And I think you said you're going to test that too. Sounds interesting. And then I see the disinfectant where it knocks it out in a minute. One minute. And is there a way we can do something like that, by injection inside or almost a cleaning because you know it gets in the lungs and does a tremendous number on the lungs? So, it'd be interesting to check that. You're going to have to use medical doctors, but it sounds interesting to me.'

Pointing a finger at his temple, Trump added: 'I'm not a doctor. But I'm, like, a person that has a good you-know-what.' He also said using 'the heat and the light' to treat the virus was 'a great thing to look at'.

The backlash from the medical profession was immediate. Pulmonologist John Balmes told Bloomberg News that 'inhaling chlorine bleach would be absolutely the worst thing for the lungs. The airway and lungs are not made to be exposed to even an aerosol of disinfectant. Not even a low dilution of bleach or isopropyl alcohol is safe. It's a totally ridiculous concept.'

Another pulmonologist Dr Vin Gupta said 'injecting or ingesting any type of cleansing product into the body is irresponsible and it's dangerous. It's a common method that people utilise when they want to kill themselves.'

Kashif Mahmood, a West Virginia doctor, warned: 'Don't take medical advice from Trump. As a physician, I can't recommend injecting disinfectant into the lungs or using UV radiation inside the body to treat COVID-19.'

It wasn't just doctors who were worried about 'Dr' Trump's crackpot theories; his own government's US Food and Drug Administration warned on its website about the dangers of a 'Miracle Mineral Solution' – basically bleach – that was being touted as a remedy for autism, cancer, HIV/AIDS, hepatitis, flu and other conditions.

'Websites selling Miracle Mineral Solution describe the product as a liquid that is 28 per cent sodium chlorite in distilled water,' says the FDA. 'Product directions instruct people to mix the sodium chlorite solution with a citric acid, such as lemon or lime juice, or another acid before drinking. In many instances, the sodium chlorite is sold with a citric acid 'activator'. When the acid is added, the mixture becomes chlorine dioxide, a powerful bleaching agent. Both sodium chlorite and chlorine dioxide are the active ingredients in disinfectants and have additional industrial uses. They are not meant to be swallowed by people...

'The FDA has received reports of consumers who have suffered from severe vomiting, severe diarrhoea, life-threatening low blood pressure caused by dehydration, and acute liver failure after drinking these products.'

The following month, Trump was again setting the medical profession's teeth on edge by announcing that he had been taking the malarial drug hydroxychloroquine, a derivative of chloroquine, for over a week in a bid to stave off the virus. 'I happen to be taking it,' he said during a White House event for restaurant executives on 18 May 2020. 'A lot of good things have come out. You'd be surprised at how many people are taking it, especially the front-line workers. Before you catch it. The front-line workers, many, many are taking it.'

Trump added: 'I'm taking it, hydroxychloroquine. Right now, yeah. Couple of weeks ago, I started taking it. Cause I think it's good, I've heard a lot of good stories.'

In sensationalist fashion, he went so far as to say the drug could become 'one of the biggest game changers in the history of medicine'.

The drug was not new. As well as malaria, it was also used at the time to treat lupus and rheumatoid arthritis, but it wasn't proven to be effective for COVID-19. A few days earlier, the FDA had warned that hydroxychloroquine, taken in combination with the antibiotic azithromycin, had caused 'serious heart rhythm problems' in patients who had tried using it for COVID. The warning referenced a Brazilian study into the drug's effects on coronavirus that was halted for safety reasons after volunteers developed irregular heart rates that caused fatal heart attacks.

About half of the eighty-one coronavirus patients in the study who lived in the city of Manaus in the Amazon were given a low dose of 450 milligrams of chloroquine for five days, with two doses on the first day. The others were prescribed a high dose of 600 milligrams twice daily for ten days.

In less than three days, the patients on the higher doses were suffering from heart arrhythmias and by the eleventh day, six of the volunteers were dead, prompting the testing to be abandoned.

'To me, this study conveys one useful piece of information, which is that chloroquine causes a dose-dependent increase in an abnormality in the ECG that could predispose people to sudden cardiac death,' Dr David Juurlink, an internist and the head of the division of clinical pharmacology at the University of Toronto, told the *New York Times*.

Some doctors also associated the drug with suicidal behaviour.

Unbowed, Trump said he would continue taking the drug. 'I'm not going to get hurt by it. It's been around for forty years. For malaria, for lupus, for other things,' he said. 'I take it. Front-line workers take it. A lot of doctors take it – excuse me, a lot of doctors take it. I take it.'

He insisted his only motive was for 'the people of this nation to feel good'.

'I don't want them feeling sick. And there's a very good

chance that this has an impact, especially early on. I take a pill every day. At some point I'll stop. What I'd like to do is, I'd like to have the cure and/or the vaccine and that'll happen I think very soon.

'It seems to have an impact, and maybe it does, maybe it doesn't,' he added. 'But if it doesn't, you're not going to get sick or die. This is a pill that's been used for a long time, for thirty, forty years.'

If his intention was to persuade the public to follow his lead, it certainly worked. The president's remarks sparked an unprecedented demand for hydroxychloroquine and chloroquine which, while still unsanctioned by the FDA, could legally be prescribed 'off label' by doctors, often under the brand name Plaquenil.

Among the consequences listed by Science.org were panic buying around the world, shortages of the drug for lupus and rheumatoid arthritis patients, a ban on exports from India, one of the world's biggest manufacturers, and a number of deaths, including a series of suicides in Nigeria and one Arizona man who self-dosed with a toxic version of chloroquine used to clean fish tanks. One patient in Wuhan ordered a small dose of 1.8 grams online and ended up in intensive care with a malignant cardiac arrhythmia.

One desperate patient tweeted: 'lupus patients like myself need help. Pharmacies are out of stock of Plaquenil. I personally called dozens of pharmacies in NYC and had friends calling in Boston. This is endangering lives.'

Interest in the treatment began with a tweet from Tesla founder Elon Musk including a link to apparent successes chloroquine had shown in early trials in France and China. 'Maybe worth considering chloroquine for C19,' he wrote.

The tweet was picked up by a few right-wing media networks, including Fox News. From there it was a short hop to Trump, who devoured the twenty-four-hour conservative news network from his quarters in the West Wing.

In turn, Trump gushed over the drug, believing it to have real possibilities as a silver bullet to end the pandemic. He told reporters at a press briefing about one man's miraculous recovery. 'They had given him the drug just a little while before, but he thought it was over,' said Trump. 'His family thought he was going to die. A number of hours later, he woke up, felt good ... He's in good shape. And he's very happy for this particular drug that we got approved in record-setting time. There's never been anything even close to it.'

However, it turned out that a study that Fox's Tucker Carlson had espoused as having 100 per cent cure rate was, in fact, a preliminary report using just twenty patients, way too few for any realistic projections.

As question marks grew over the drug and it became clear it wasn't changing any games, Trump backed away from it. And then he caught COVID.

CHAPTER 13:

THE QANON SHAMAN AND A CULT THAT LOOKS LIKE YOU
– 6 January 2021

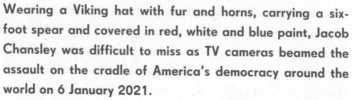

Wearing a Viking hat with fur and horns, carrying a six-foot spear and covered in red, white and blue paint, Jacob Chansley was difficult to miss as TV cameras beamed the assault on the cradle of America's democracy around the world on 6 January 2021.

Chansley was among the first thirty rioters to enter the United States Capitol as the votes were being counted to confirm Joe Biden as America's forty-sixth president. Shirtless and carrying a giant bullhorn, he led the interlopers past the flimsy police lines and into the scaffolding erected in readiness for Biden's upcoming inauguration on top of the staircase leading up to the Lower West Terrace.

At 2:10pm, with the unwitting lawmakers still verifying the election votes in the chamber under the watchful eye of Vice President Mike Pence, the rioters burst on to the Upper West Terrace and broke through a door to get inside the building. With security staff caught by surprise, Chansley kept going through into the Senate Chamber and headed straight to the dais on the Senate floor where Pence had been sitting just minutes before.

Taking selfies as he sat in Pence's chair, the bearded Trump supporter scribbled on a piece of paper, 'It's only a matter of time. Justice is coming!' and led chants over his bullhorn before finally being forced from the rotunda at 3:09pm.

It was no great surprise when the FBI came knocking on his door in Phoenix, Arizona just three days later. He was, after all, the most instantly recognisable rioter. But few people would recognise Chansley by his real name, even after he was jailed for forty-one months on 17 November 2021 for his part in the riot.

He was much better known as the QAnon shaman.

The storming of the Capitol was just the latest high-profile incident involving the shadowy conspiracy theory group that was making concrete inroads into America's seats of power. Less flamboyant but equally committed QAnon supporters were spotted inside the Capitol and in the crowds outside, some carrying banners with the group's slogan, 'Follow the white rabbit'.

If the QAnon Shaman could be dismissed as a self-promoting showman, some of the group's other leading figures were forcing the nation's ruling elite to take them seriously because of the scale of their support from the extreme right wing given a voice by Donald Trump. One outspoken QAnon supporter was even voted into US Congress, the equivalent of winning a seat as a Member of Parliament. While not endorsing QAnon, the former president has described its followers as 'people who love our country'. Asked to disassociate himself with the group at a town hall question and answer session in 2020, Trump initially said he knew 'nothing about QAnon', but added, 'I do know that they are very much against paedophilia, and I agree with that.'

This may come as no surprise as Trump tends to like people who hero worship him and QAnon certainly loves Trump, espousing a bizarre, utterly unfounded theory that he is fighting a secret battle against Satan-worshipping Democrat paedophiles in government, Hollywood and the media that will one day come to a day of reckoning when they will be arrested and executed.

Believers claim that Joe Biden, Hillary Clinton and Barack Obama are members of this 'deep state' cabal, as well as entertainers such as Oprah Winfrey, Tom Hanks and Ellen DeGeneres, and religious leaders like the Pope and the Dalai Lama. QAnon says these prominent people kill and eat their victims to get a chemical called adrenochrome that is supposed to help them live longer lives.

The group's origins date back to 2017 and an anonymous social media user calling themselves the 'Q Clearance Patriot' who wrote a series of posts on the toxic '4chan' message board, a fringe platform often used by online extremists. The 'Q' was supposed to be a reference to a high-security government and offer a spurious authority to the posts, which suggested 'The Storm' was approaching when Trump would move against the Satanic paedophiles and make America great again. 'The Storm' was a reference to a remark Trump made to his military chiefs at a 2017 photo op when he said: 'You guys know what this represents? Maybe it's the calm before the storm.'

Q's identity is unknown, but he/they have posted more than 5,000 cryptic messages, known to QAnon followers as 'drops' on a series of message boards, including '8chan' and '8kun' as well as '4chan'. These drops use codes for some of their recurring characters, including POTUS for Trump, BC for Bill Clinton, HRC for Hillary Clinton and HUSSEIN for Barack Obama.

While Facebook, YouTube and Twitter have all blocked

QAnon content, its scope and variety makes it impossible to control. For example, QAnon supporters hijacked the hashtag for a 2020 'Save the Children' campaign by a legitimate anti-child trafficking group and used it to spread its own theories.

How many people believe this crazy stuff, you might ask? The answer is a hell of a lot more people than you would imagine. NBC reported that an internal Facebook investigation uncovered thousands of QAnon-linked groups and pages – with more than three million members and followers.

QAnon started out as a uniquely American concept with a domestic cast of characters and Trumpian goals. But the COVID pandemic was perfectly timed for the very twenty-first century conspiracy theory to spread across the Atlantic to the disenfranchised looking for alternative populist answers to what they saw as increasingly overreaching governments. They saw QAnon as a call to arms over COVID-19. Conspiracy theories abounded under the umbrella of a group of like-minded believers. People were stuck at home, isolated, worried and many of them living in an online bubble.

In October 2020, the *Guardian* carried the results of a survey that claimed one in four Britons agreed with QAnon conspiracies. Researchers for the organisation Hope Not Hate reported that 17 per cent of those questioned believed that COVID was spread on purpose by the United Nations as part of a 'depopulation plan' to create a 'new world order'.

Young people were particularly partial to conspiracies. Just 6 per cent said they supported QAnon, but 25 per cent believed that 'secret Satanic cults exist and include influential elites'. For people aged between eighteen and twenty-four, that percentage rose to 38 per cent.

Of the twenty-five- to thirty-four-year-olds questioned, 42

per cent believed there was 'a single group of people who secretly control events and rule the world together'.

'The incorporation of COVID-19 conspiracy theories into the QAnon narrative has the potential to erode trust in medical experts and authorities, and further the spread of health misinformation and pseudoscience in the midst of a global pandemic,' said Hope Not Hate.

David Lawrence, a researcher with Hope Not Hate, told the BBC: 'Public trust in institutions has declined in the UK in recent years, and has been exacerbated by the handling of the pandemic. This has provided ideal conditions for conspiracy theories to spread.'

In late August 2020, a group protesting child abuse marched through Central London and ended up outside Buckingham Palace where, to the bemusement of sightseers and to people watching on the TV news, the protesters from 'Freedom for the Children UK' shouted 'paedophile' towards the royal residence. The slur was a sign that QAnon's campaign against the elites, the establishment, was taking root in Britain.

However, the ethnically diverse group was peculiarly British and fuelled by the lockdown that had forced the nation inside in a bid to control the rampaging virus. The London march comprised of mainly young people and women, many with children, and led by two women, Laura Ward and Lucy Davis. Similar rallies took place across the UK, including Manchester, Bristol and Birmingham.

The following month, the same group held an even bigger protest marching from Oxford Street to Parliament Square. Again, women and children were prominent. Onlookers may have been confused at the cryptic initials 'WWG1WGA' on the T-shirts of some of the young marchers. They stood for 'Where We Go One,

We Go All,' a line from the 1996 Jeff Bridges film *White Squall* misattributed by QAnon to President John F. Kennedy and one of the group's not-so-secretive slogans. Other slogans on T-shirts and placards referred to 'Pizzagate', a favourite QAnon conspiracy involving Hillary Clinton, suggesting the former First Lady ran a child sex ring out of a Washington restaurant, and popular 'Q' terms such as 'spirit cooking', 'frazzledrip', 'dark to light', 'adrenochrome' and 'paedogate'. Pandemic Britain was a breeding ground for QAnon, even if the march organisers insisted there was no direct connection.

Unlike in America, supporters weren't necessarily right-leaning – Q-related posts were found among pro and anti-conservative groups. Nevertheless, Britain quickly became the biggest pool of QAnon support outside the US, according to BBC researchers. In the three months leading up to 13 October 2020, their analysis, based on data from CrowdTangle and Spredfast, found that the innocuous-sounding #SaveTheChildren and #SaveOurChildren hashtags hijacked by QAnon were used 1.5 million times on Twitter and triggered over 28 million interactions on Facebook and Instagram. The UK was more active in QAnon circles than any other European country, including Germany, France and the Netherlands where the movement was growing.

QAnon videos with titles like 'Murder By 'Vaccine' – The Evidence Mounts!' and 'Doctors and Nurses Giving the Coronavirus Vaccine Will Be Tried as War Criminals' have been viewed tens of thousands of times. Their biggest target was vaccines, saying, for example, they alter the DNA and represent the biblical 'mark of the beast'.

Nick Backovic, a contributing editor at Logically, told the BBC that the UK demographic for the QAnon-related marches did not follow the far-right stereotype. 'These weren't your typically "red-pilled" conspiracy theorists,' he said. 'They were worried mums and dads who had been scared into believing these exaggerated stats that aren't backed up by any evidence.'

Cults and conspiracy theories have always flourished during times of upheaval and crisis and the confusing and chaotic information during the pandemic left many, even the most subservient, questioning the decisions of their leaders. How can you follow the science when scientists have so many conflicting opinions? How can you trust a government narrative that is constantly changing on a dime? Why should we follow rules that plainly make no common sense? The debacle over Christmas parties at 10 Downing Street while the rest of the nation was in lockdown and the prime minister's top aides ignoring their own laws further fuel the unrest. Amidst this confusion and distrust, people feeling isolated from their families and neighbours – both physically and emotionally – are finding like-minded communities through social media and QAnon followers no longer look like land-locked Viking Jacob Chansley with his bullish bullhorn.

They look like you and me and whisper to millions online.

CHAPTER 14:

DRASTIC ACTION REQUIRED
– 18 May 2020

▼

The line-up of the whistle-blower media team behind the most effective investigations into the origins of the COVID pandemic looks more like the cast of a video game with names like The Seeker, Sherlock G. Nomes, Citizen 'O', Galileo Principle, Rads, Lab Leak and Citizen Dot Matrix. Together, they have a name straight out of a Marvel superhero movie – D.R.A.S.T.I.C. They aren't journalists or scientists or detectives. They are the new breed of citizen reporters with no agenda except to get to the truth. They usually work in a publicity vacuum, spending countless hours in front of their computer screens trying to solve problems that paid employees simply do not have time to pursue.

It is a relatively new phenomenon where laypeople have the interest and determination to delve into the labyrinth of the internet and discover information that journalists, scientists and detectives have not or could not find. Most of the time these people work on the fringes and the facts they find are for their own interest or that of their immediate circles. Occasionally, they will come out into the open, such as during the missing person case that gripped America in the summer of 2021 when a young woman, Gabby Petito, disappeared while on a 'van life' trip across the country with her boyfriend Brian Laundrie. Suspicions were raised when Laundrie returned home to Florida without his girlfriend. Eventually, Petito's body was found and Laundrie, who is believed to have killed her, committed suicide but the clues to find the missing woman – and her killer boyfriend – came not from the detectives on the case but largely from people online who were invested in the search and uncovered information the police had neither the time nor the expertise to find.

COVID was an even bigger case with a great deal more at stake and, once more, the traditional investigators, the Fourth Estate, wasn't up to the job. It was too slow, too biased, whether right or left, too encumbered, and too entitled. Donald Trump's xenophobia had thrown up a barrier that made it unseemly to believe the Chinese could be to blame, either for some kind of lab leak or just for covering up the crisis. It was deemed another Trump/Fox News tirade and unworthy of most of the mainstream media. They simply stopped looking.

But D.R.A.S.T.I.C. (Decentralized Radical Autonomous Search Team Investigating COVID-19), this group of committed amateurs with cartoonish avatars, kept searching the Internet for the holy grail of how it started. It should have been ground zero for any probe into the pandemic, but it was left to about two dozen loosely aligned people working independently from a series of different countries to work it out for themselves.

In the end, they built up a database of so much circumstantial evidence – including details of the 2012 Yunnan mineshaft outbreak – that even President Joe Biden couldn't ignore it. Only when the White House made a surprise announcement that the intelligence services were finally investigating the lab leak theory did the traditional media finally wake up to the story.

As *Newsweek* put it, these web detectives uncovered obscure documents, pieced together information, and explained it in meticulous detail on long Twitter threads – 'in a kind of open-source, collective brainstorming session that was part forensic science, part citizen journalism, and entirely new.'

Their success wasn't overnight, nor was it simple. Rossana Segreto, a microbiologist at Austria's University of Innsbruck, discovered the first piece of the puzzle with an apparent oversight, conscious or otherwise, by Wuhan's 'Bat Woman' Zhengli Shi. Shi's infamous 3 February 2020 report published in *Nature* revealed that the bat coronavirus RaTG13 was the closest relative to SARS-CoV-2, or COVID-19, without actually saying the sample came from the Yunnan mineshaft or its human cost.

Two days later, a second paper claimed that a bat sample fragment – BtCov/4991 – found by Shi and her team in an abandoned mineshaft in Yunnan Province in 2013 was an even closer relative. Suspicious about the similarities in the stories, Segreto checked out whether 4991 matched any other known viruses using an online search tool called BLAST, a kind of Google for viruses, and found it was a 100 per cent match for RaTG13. They were one and the same virus.

What started out as a nerdy escapade to see what they could dig up took on a heightened significance from 18 May 2020 when another member of the team, a former science teacher in India known only as 'The Seeker', was sifting through a Chinese scientific database when he stumbled upon a master's thesis, written by a Chinese doctor, that described in detail how the six miners clearing up bat faeces in the Yunnan copper mine fell suddenly sick with a SARS-like virus in 2012. That thesis provided the basis for much of the breakthrough information I included in Chapter 1. The Seeker was also able to confirm that bats from that same mine had been sampled by the Wuhan Institute of Virology. He had found a 1,000-mile bridge linking RaTG13, if not COVID-19 itself, all the way from the Yunnan bat cave where six miners fell terribly sick in 2012 to the Institute of Virology right in the epicentre of the 2019–20 pandemic.

'Finding it, at that moment, felt big, like a homicide detective solving a cold case,' The Seeker told CNET. Suddenly there was an alternative narrative to the convenient conjecture that the wet market in Wuhan was to blame. The master's thesis, as we have already learned, certainly contradicted Shi's later claims that the miners died from a fungal infection. Together with the information dug up by Segreto, gaping holes were beginning to appear in the accepted story of the virus's origins. By this time, Facebook was flagging up such online conversations as 'false information' and most of D.R.A.S.T.I.C.'s discourse took place on Twitter. The group was pulled together by someone going under the fake name of Billy Bostickson and now has more than twenty-eight members, about half of whom remain anonymous. Their direct approach has not always been appreciated by scientists who, more cautious by profession, have been sceptical about some half-cocked views that haven't come near to any peer review process. But D.R.A.S.T.I.C. has undoubtedly been instrumental in bringing the debate back out into the open and has led calls for the World Health Organization to reopen its flawed probe into the source of the pandemic. As David Asher, an ex-State Department investigator told *Vanity*

Fair: 'The DRASTIC people are doing better research than the US government.' The WHO's widely panned first report into its cursory investigation into the origin of the pandemic was published in late March of 2021. The joint international team comprised of seventeen Chinese and seventeen international experts who spent twenty-eight days between 14 January and 10 February in Wuhan trying to work out what happened. They didn't do a very good job.

Apparently ignoring stories like that of English language teacher Connor Reed and the *South China Morning Post*'s reliable reporting, the WHO wrote off claims that COVID was already in Wuhan during October and November 2019, despite confirming there were 76,253 'records of cases of respiratory conditions' in those two months.

'Although ninety-two cases were considered to be compatible with SARS-CoV-2 infection after review, subsequent testing and further external multidisciplinary clinical review determined that none was in fact due to SARS-CoV-2 infection,' said the report, continuing: 'Based on the analysis of this and other surveillance data, it is considered unlikely that any substantial transmission of SARS-CoV-2 infection was occurring in Wuhan during those two months.'

Its findings, in short, were that:

Direct zoonotic spillover is considered to be a possible-to-likely pathway.

Introduction through an intermediate host is considered to be a likely to very likely pathway.

Introduction through cold/ food chain products is considered a possible pathway.

Introduction through a laboratory incident was considered to be an extremely unlikely pathway.

The blowback from the report came fast and furious. The 'possible pathway' involving the virus being imported into China on frozen food was Beijing's favourite theory but widely disregarded by experts.

The lab leak theory was apparently dismissed out of hand with the WHO team recommending it need no longer be investigated, a proposal which, by that time, seemed out of step with emerging expert opinion. Even critics were open to the theory being thoroughly looked at. Many felt the report stunk of a cover-up.

At the press conference announcing the report's publication, WHO Director-General Tedros Adhanom Ghebreyesus was stepping back the lab leak snub, suggesting the theory required further attention.

'Although the team has concluded that a laboratory leak is the least likely hypothesis, this requires further investigation, potentially with additional missions involving specialist experts, which I am ready to deploy,' he said.

D.R.A.S.T.I.C.'s Billy Bostickson published an open letter to ten international members of the WHO COVID-19 investigation team – Prof. John Watson (Public Health England, United Kingdom), Prof. Dr Thea Fisher, MD, DMSc (PhD) (Nordsjællands Hospital, Denmark), Prof. Dr Marion Koopmans, DVM PhD (Erasmus MC, Netherlands), Prof. Dr Dominic Dwyer, MD (Westmead Hospital, Australia), Vladimir Dedkov, Ph.D (Institut Pasteur, Russia), Dr Hung Nguyen, PhD (International Livestock Research Institute (ILRI), Vietnam), PD. Dr med vet. Fabian Lendertz (Robert Koch-Institute, Germany), Dr Peter Daszak, Ph.D (EcoHealth Alliance, USA), Dr Farag El Moubasher, Ph.D (Ministry of Public Health, Qatar) and Prof. Dr Ken Maeda, PhD, DVM (National Institute of Infectious Diseases, Japan).

Dear Fellow Scientists,

The COVID-19 pandemic has been ravaging the world for over a year now and it is showing no sign of easing in many countries, with infection cases and death tolls continuing to climb. Millions of our brothers and sisters have lost their loved ones, their jobs, businesses, livelihoods and education opportunities. The economies of many nations have been severely compromised, resulting in great tribulation for many sectors, with many closed or bankrupt businesses and millions of unemployed.

Sadly today, we are all still as much in the dark as to the origins of COVID-19 as we were ten months ago, despite numerous scientific studies and research conducted around the world since then.

We are glad that the WHO is able to form an investigation team of ten international experts sitting in the East to undertake the task of unravelling these mysteries and take us from darkness to light.

We, the concerned people around the world, on behalf of all those who have died, widowers, widows, distressed sons, daughters and orphans, therefore call on you to conduct the investigation with transparency, impartiality and bravery without bowing to any pressure or national interest.

Such an investigation, to be both credible and successful must take into consideration all scenarios in a scientific way without giving preference to any default hypothesis, however disturbing this may be.

In support of this investigation, a dedicated group of researchers in various parts of the world have spent months unearthing documents, web pages, papers, and reports to compile a list of relevant and as yet unanswered questions about the origins of COVID-19.

We therefore call on the WHO investigation team to answer the following questions which we feel are of paramount importance to a successful investigation into the origins of SARS-COV-2.

We wish you success and thank you sincerely for your endeavours in search of the truth!

From Concerned People of the World

The ensuing fifty questions range from whether the WHO team has any plans for a more comprehensive visit to Shi's lab at the Institute of Virology to why its databases are still offline to asking if any of them speak Mandarin.

D.R.A.S.T.I.C. was especially interested in the 2012 Tongguan mineshaft outbreak, asking the WHO to clarify with the Wuhan Institute of Virology what happened to samples from the miners and the bats collected from the cave between 2012 and 2019 and whether they were available for independent analysis. They also wanted to know if the WIV cultured 'any virus from the Tongguan mineshaft pneumonia cases in animals or cell lines? If so, were the sequences used as "backbones" for creating other viruses?'

Unsurprisingly, they are still waiting for answers.

About the same time on 4 March 2021, a group of two dozen international scientists wrote their own open letter to the WHO demanding a new inquiry into COVID's origins, claiming the initial WHO probe earlier that year had 'insufficient access' to be credible. It was the clearest signal yet that more than a year after the outbreak began, the world's brightest minds were still in the dark.

This letter was also co-organised by another active member of D.R.A.S.T.I.C., Gilles Demaneuf, a data scientist from New Zealand.

Based on our analysis, and as confirmed by the global study convened by the World Health Organization (WHO) and Chinese authorities, there is as yet no evidence demonstrating a fully natural origin of this virus.

The zoonosis hypothesis, largely based on patterns of previous zoonosis events, is only one of a number of possible SARS-CoV-2 origins, alongside the research-related accident hypothesis. Although the 'collaborative' process of discovery mandated by the World Health Assembly in May 2020 was meant to enable a full examination of the origins of the pandemic, we believe that structural limitations built into this endeavor make it all but impossible for the WHO-convened mission to realize this aspiration.

In particular, we wish to raise public awareness of the fact that half of the joint team convened under that process is made of Chinese citizens whose scientific independence may be limited, that international members of the joint team had to rely on information the Chinese authorities chose to share with them, and that any joint team report must be approved by both the Chinese and international members of the joint team. We have therefore reached the conclusion that the joint team did not have the mandate, the independence, or the necessary accesses to carry out a full and unrestricted investigation into all the relevant SARS-CoV-2 origin hypotheses – whether natural spillover or laboratory/research related incident.

The tide was turning. In a documentary that aired on Danish television in August 2021, the expert who led the WHO mission to Wuhan, Peter Ben Embarek, said Chinese members of the team tried to prevent any mention of the possibility of a lab leak in the final report.

'In the beginning, they didn't want anything about the lab [in the report], because it was impossible, so there was no need to waste time on that,' Ben Embarek said in the interview, according to the *Washington Post*. 'We insisted on including it, because it was part of the whole issue about where the virus originated.'

The dispute reportedly lasted forty-eight hours, with the Chinese finally allowing the lab leak to be mentioned 'on the condition we didn't recommend any specific studies to further that hypothesis', he added.

Although the final wording in the report said it was 'extremely unlikely' that a lab leak was to blame, Ben Embarek said that didn't mean it was impossible. 'A lab employee infected in the field while collecting samples in a bat cave – such a scenario belongs both as a lab-leak hypothesis and as our first hypothesis of direct infection from bat to human. We've seen that hypothesis as a likely hypothesis,' the *Post* quoted him as saying in the documentary.

Does that mean a Chinese researcher who took bat samples from the Tongguan cave could have been the cause? It seems the WHO was open to the possibility after all.

The Danish TV channel said Ben Embarek suggested the Chinese authorities wouldn't want to acknowledge there might have been 'human error' involved. 'It probably means there's a human error behind such an event, and they're not very happy to admit that,' he was quoted as saying. 'The whole system focuses a lot on being infallible, and everything must be perfect. Somebody could also wish to hide something. Who knows?'

It seems certain the international members of the investigative team had been under enormous pressure from their Chinese colleagues and from health officials. 'The politics was always in the room with us on the other side of the table,' Ben Embarek told *Science* magazine earlier in 2021.

Soon the US government was also questioning the independence of the report.. 'We have deep concerns about the way in which the early findings of the COVID-19 investigation were communicated and questions about the underlying process used to reach them,' said State Department spokesman Ned Price. 'It's imperative that this report be independent, with expert findings free from intervention or alteration by Chinese government authorities in order to better understand this pandemic and prepare for the next one.'

It didn't help the Chinese that the state media had hitched on to a Facebook post by a 'Swiss biologist' named Wilson Edwards who complained the US was politicising the probe into the pandemic's origins. 'The US is so obsessed with attacking China on the origin-tracing issue that it is reluctant to open its eyes to the data and findings,' he charged in the post, which was exploited by Chinese state media to vindicate Beijing's stance on soft-peddling the report.

The only problem was that Mr Edwards didn't appear to exist.

'Looking for Wilson Edwards, alleged biologist, cited in press and social media in China over the last several days,' the Swiss Embassy in Beijing tweeted on 10 August 2021. 'If you exist, we would like to meet you! But it is more likely that this is a fake news, and we call on the Chinese press and netizens to take down the posts.'

It was one of the easier theories to debunk. The Chinese media took down the stories. Without correction.

CHAPTER 15:

BILL GATES & PHISH AND CHIPS
– 19 March 2020

Victims of conspiracy theories face a dilemma whether they are ordinary folks or the richest human in the world. By ignoring the stories about them can mean speculation grows online until they are accepted as facts by many people. By denying them, the victim gives the claims legitimacy, however spurious they may be, and bring them out of the darker web and into the open.

'Well, he/she would say that wouldn't they,' is the usual retort to attempts by the subjects of conspiracy theories to go public with their disclaimers.

Bill Gates has good reason to expect some gratitude for the nearly $2 billion he has pledged to global efforts to combat coronavirus. The Bill and Melinda Gates Foundation may well have saved more lives in the pandemic than any other private institution. But having that much money and power brings with it a unique set of issues; people tend to distrust your motives.

So, while Gates and his foundation have the best of intentions in trying to save the world from COVID-19, conspiracy theorists, many of them ordinary individuals without any connection to organised activist groups, believe he's pushing vaccines to implant microchips in a Dr Evil plot to control billions of unwitting people.

Gates never expected such widespread attacks. 'I'm surprised at all the conspiracy theories – people who think the vaccine is not meant to save lives,' he told attendees at the World Congress of Science & Factual Producers in December 2020. 'That's all wrong, but the scale of it is a bit scary in terms of, will that prevent people from being willing to take the vaccine, and why are they looking for these simple explanations?'

'It's almost hard to deny this stuff because it's so stupid or strange that even to repeat it gives it credibility,' he told Reuters news agency in January 2021. 'We're really going to have to get educated about this over the next year and understand ... how does it change people's behaviour and how should we have minimised this?'

'But,' he added, 'do people really believe that stuff?'

I hate to tell you this, Bill, but yes. They do.

A typical Facebook post at the height of the pandemic (with 22,000 shares) read: 'Gates wants us microchipped and Fauci wants us to carry vax certificates,' referring to Bill Gates and Anthony Fauci, Chief Medical Advisor to the President of the United States. Another post (with 51,000 shares) read: 'Due to the large number of people who will refuse the forthcoming COVID-19 vaccine because it will include tracking microchips, the Gates Foundation is now spending billions of dollars to ensure that all medical and dental injections and procedures include the chips so that the only way to avoid being 'chipped' will be to refuse any and all dental and medical treatment. Please repost this information in as many media as possible to help this important warning to go viral. They will not be allowed to pull the wool over our eyes if freedom loving independent thinkers everywhere stand up to them and make the world aware of this scheme.'

These messages have either been deleted or flagged up by Facebook as containing false information – and denied emphatically by Gates and the foundation – but a quick look through the threads shows these people are far from alone and far from the most extreme. And while some of the facts they are based on may seem surreal, the consequences are very real.

The Bill Gates microchip theory is the most viral conspiracy theory of the pandemic – a poll by *The Economist* and YouGov found that half of all Americans refusing the COVID vaccine bought into the fake theory and the Microsoft founder has been forced to admit the result has been that fewer people have been vaccinated than he expected.

A survey published by the Kaiser Family Foundation found that 78 per cent of US adults either believed at least one item of misinformation about COVID or vaccines or were unsure whether the misinformation was true or false. Another poll, this time commissioned by Yahoo News and YouGov, found that 44 per cent of Republicans and 19 per cent of Democrats believed Gates was secretly planning to implant microchips in billions of people.

The billionaire has also had to fend off baseless claims that he developed the virus in a lab to kill off 15 per cent of the world's population; that his foundation tested vaccines on 'guinea pig' children in India and Africa, leading to thousands of deaths and injuries; and that a tetanus vaccine he introduced in Kenya included abortion drugs.

In a blog post in December 2021, Gates confessed one of his biggest concerns is in 'finding ways to combat disinformation'.

He continued: 'I thought demand for vaccines would be way higher than it has been in places like the United States. It's clear that disinformation (including conspiracy theories that unfortunately involve me) is having a substantial impact on people's willingness to get vaccinated. This is part of a larger trend toward distrust in institutions, and it's one of the issues I'm most worried about heading into 2022.'

The microchip theories were fuelled by some of the usual suspects. Never a regime to miss an opportunity to sow mistrust of the West online, the Russians were all over it. The leader of Russia's Communist Party Gennady Zyuganov launched a tirade against 'capitalist globalism' in a column. While not naming Gates, he claimed 'globalists are ready to use the most sophisticated technologies of digital enslavement. Among them is the unspoken mass chipization, which they may eventually resort to under the pretext of mandatory vaccination against coronavirus. The ideologues of digital fascism have allies among the owners of the largest corporations, bank executives and high-ranking officials – including in our country.' More bizarrely, Trump's long-time friend and advisor Roger Stone told right-wing talk show host Joe Piscopo in April 2020 that Gates could have played a part in creating the virus for his own nefarious ends. 'Whether Bill Gates played some role in the creation and spread of this virus is open for vigorous debate,' he said. 'I have conservative friends who say it's ridiculous and others say absolutely. He and other globalists are using it for mandatory vaccinations and microchipping people so we know if they've been tested. Over my dead body. Mandatory vaccinations? No way, José!'

Stone was convicted of impeding a congressional probe into Trump's 2016 White House campaign and possible ties to Russia and convicted of forty months in prison before being pardoned by Trump on 23 December 2020, just as the virus was gathering momentum in Wuhan.

Like most theories, there's a seed of a story that germinates online. In Gates' case, the idea that he wants to microchip everybody stems from a 2019 experiment by researchers from MIT in Massachusetts investigating whether an invisible dye that would become visible on the skin using a smartphone app could be used to show whether someone is vaccinated or not. This was clearly before the pandemic hit but it hit, a chord with anti-vaxxers because it was funded in part by the Bill and Melinda Gates Foundation (along with the National Science Foundation, the US Department of Energy, the National Institute of Biomedical Imaging and Bioengineering, the National Natural Science Foundation of China and the Youth Innovation Promotion Association).

The MIT report, published in *Science* on 18 December 2019, showed how the researchers injected 'biocompatible, near-infrared quantum dots' that are invisible to the naked eye into the skin with 'dissolvable microneedles that deliver patterns of near-infrared light-emitting microparticles to the skin.' It continued: 'Particle patterns are invisible to the eye but can be imaged using modified smartphones. By co-delivering a vaccine, the pattern of particles in the skin could serve as an on-person vaccination record.'

The technique was tested on rats but never got any further. Unless, of course, you believe the conspiracy theorists. Perhaps the most rapacious of conspiracy theorists may have missed this relatively minor research project. After all, Kevin McHugh, one of the lead authors, confirmed there was never a plan to insert a microchip or any kind of mini capsule under the human skin; it was more like an invisible tattoo. But then Bill Gates himself referred to it and the floodgates opened. He didn't even refer directly to the dot dye research and his apparently innocent remark was buried halfway down a 19 March 2020 'Gates Notes' blog running through his answers to questions he was asked about COVID on Reddit the previous day.

'Eventually we will have some digital certificates to show who has recovered or been tested recently or when we have a vaccine who has received it,' he replied to a question about how to keep businesses running during the pandemic. He wasn't even talking about microchips but about an open-source digital platform to expand home-based COVID testing. It didn't really matter what he meant. It didn't matter that the smallest type of 5G chip that could be manufactured was the size of a penny and way too big to fit in any needle. The misinformation machine was up and running.

One typical tweet included a photo of the back of a man's bald head with a barcode across it and the caption: 'Bill Gates is launching implantable chips which will be used to show whether a person has been tested and vaccinated for Corona. These microchips will dissolve under the skin, leaving identification "quantum dots". These implants can also be used as a form of ID.'

It got so bad in America the Rhode Island Department of Health felt compelled to tweet: 'Despite what you may have heard, COVID-19 vaccines will not change your personality, make you grow a third eye, or alter your DNA. They are definitely microchip-free. @VaccinateyourFamily.'

Still, take the fact that Gates has spent countless millions on improving the ways that vaccinations are delivered, particularly to Third World countries where record-keeping may not be as effective as elsewhere, add an experiment with invisible 'ink' and a liberal dose of paranoia and you can come up with one of the world's richest men with a secret plot to give everyone a chip on their shoulder.

James Tabery, a professor at the University of Utah with a special interest in history and the philosophy of science and bioethics, says people in the public eye such as Gates, Fauci and George Soros – another billionaire targeted by anti-vaxxers in the microchip theory – are attractive foes to conspiracy theorists.

'There's something intriguing about the possibility that these powerful people are behind the scenes or puppet masters fooling us all, and I think there's also something alluring about being on the side of really knowing what's going on ... that's attractive – the idea that you're in the know as opposed to the other people who aren't,' Tabery told ABC. 'The world is a chaotic place,' he added. 'There's a lot of strange, unpredictable, awful things that happen from tsunamis that kill a quarter of a million people to pandemics that kill more. Oftentimes conspiracy theories are about making the chaotic world seem less chaotic.

'Combatting a pandemic requires widespread community coordination and putting your individual interests in some sense – deprioritising them in the name of the public good – and all these narratives, whether it's the Bill Gates variety or the George Soros variety or the 5G towers variety, they delegitimize the official explanation which makes it less likely that somebody is going to do their part.'

Tabery says that even if a theory is proved to be false, the distrust of the official narrative remains, but he thinks it's unlikely the public will continue to wonder about the Gates microchip in the same way they do about the JFK assassination or 9/11 because it is so current; people will understand over time that they have not been chipped. 'Millions of people are being vaccinated, and you're not finding that people are being microchipped,' he said. 'There are some side effects, but it's not super dangerous ... the hope is as time goes on a lot of this stuff is going to disappear. The way you have people sixty years later wondering about the JFK assassination or still talking about the 9/11 truthers, I don't think even five years from now you're going to find a lot of people playing up the Bill Gates microchip conspiracy theory.' That may be so, but I suspect Bill Gates has forever entered the parade of famous names associated with conspiracy theories that keep coming up when people are looking with suspicion at the 'global elites'.

Another academic, Professor Joseph Uscinski, a political scientist at the University of Miami and author of *American Conspiracy Theories*, told the BBC he believes that Gates' wealth and fame are to blame for him becoming the 'voodoo doll' of conspiracy theories.'Conspiracy theories are about accusing powerful people of doing terrible things,' he said. 'The theories are basically the same, just the names change. Before Bill Gates, it was George Soros and the Koch brothers and the Rothschilds and the Rockefellers.

'It should come as no surprise that rich people and big corporations are being accused of conspiring to put chips in our necks because that is a thing we fear. This has been the ammo of conspiracy theories for a long, long time.'

As much as Gates hit back against the misinformation, with the considerable backing of his financial clout, his foundation and his influential connections, they continued to cross over into the national debate on the coronavirus, to the extent that an independent MP demanded in the Italian Parliament that he be referred to the International Criminal Court for crimes against humanity. At Trump rallies and QAnon gatherings, anti-vaxxers can often be seen carrying signs reading '#SayNoToBillGates'.

In a 9 April 2020 interview with CNBC, Gates discussed the difficulties in offering vaccines to older people, saying: 'Here, we clearly need a vaccine that works in the upper age range because they're most at risk of that. And doing that so that you amp it up so it works in older people and yet you don't have side effects ... you know, if we have one in 10,000 side effects, that's way more, 700,000 people who will suffer from that. So, really understanding the safety at gigantic scale across all age ranges – you know, pregnant, male, female, undernourished, existing comorbidities – it's very, very hard. And that actual decision of, OK, let's go and give this vaccine to the entire world – governments will have to be involved because there will be some risk and indemnification needed before that can be decided on.'

That's what Gates said. He's referring to side effects from the jabs, saying that in theory if seven billion people are vaccinated and one in ten thousand people suffer from side effects that would mean 700,000 people would suffer from them. He didn't mention anything about people dying.

It wasn't long before a twisted version of the quote was going viral. 'Bill Gates admits the vaccine will no doubt kill 700,000 people,' read a post on a UK Twitter account. '700,000 potential injuries from COVID vaccine according to Gates himself. But WHO & Big Public Health will still find a way to blame the victims,' read another post on Twitter. A German article shared 19,000 times on Facebook had the headline, 'Bill Gates predicts 700,000 victims from corona[virus] vaccination.' The article goes on: 'According to Gates, that would be 8,300 corona vaccination victims for Germany with its 83 million inhabitants. He calls this – death or permanent disability – "side effects".'

Robert Goldberg, History Professor at the University of Utah and author of *Enemies Within: The Culture of Conspiracy in Modern America*, believes trust in the motives of science has been eroded over time and the current generation is more suspicious of vaccines. 'We had no problem whatsoever because there was an absolute faith that science was doing good, but I think over the last fifty years there's been a decided change in that,' he told ABC.

'I think there is a profound distrust of American institutions and the medical profession and medicine in general and science,' he added. 'I think the idea that we have – we're going to trust science and science will protect us – is being turned on its head by people who distrust those kinds of authorities and institutions and trust those who are naysayers and who seek to discredit all of our institutions. If you have a distrust and you do have faith in the system and in the people who govern that system, the idea that people would turn events like the plague (the pandemic) for nefarious purposes is something that comes readily to their minds.' Goldberg shares my belief that COVID conspiracy theories involving 5G and Bill Gates are no longer the preserve of extremists or activists with an agenda. They are discussed over drinks at the pub or at Sunday lunch. And the distrust in the establishment was spreading even before the pandemic.'This is not simply a lunatic fringe. This is not simply the extreme,' he said in the ABC interview. 'What has happened is conspiracy thinking has breached the mainstream. It's left the banks and is now in the mainstream of American thought and opinion, and that's what the concern is. This is less fear than trust and faith, and when you don't trust your leaders and you don't trust media to give you the news, to give you the facts, you seek alternatives, you seek counter authorities. And that's where those conspiracy theories blossom and bloom. 'What these conspiracy theories do is they create a world of good versus evil, or right versus wrong, and if people believe that everybody is opposed to you or disagrees with you, is a traitor, has betrayed the trust, then the very foundations of this country ... is lost and then we go into a future facing very difficult problems without that ability to solve the problems that we're going to be having to deal with.'

Some Gates baiters point to a 2015 TED talk in Vancouver, Canada, in which he warned that 'if anything kills over ten million people over the next few decades, it is likely to be a highly infectious virus, rather than a war.' Did Gates have a sinister prior knowledge that the pandemic was coming? I highly doubt it.

But then along comes another conspiracy theory involving Bill Gates and the US government that it's just too hard to resist. I mean, what are the odds of a US congressional bill about COVID being called H.R.6666? The law was passed to provide medical groups around the country doing COVID testing and contact tracing with $100 billion in emergency funding. It was also known as the TRACE Act, so it was inevitable that Gates' name would come up.

'This is what Bill Gates and George Soros want to do ... Secretly stick you with a chip while testing you for the coronavirus ... the Dems have a bill on the house floor ready to vote on it to require this ... House Bill 6666 ... no bull ... look it up and WAKE UP !!!!' read one widely shared Facebook post that was accompanied by a graphic showing a medic taking a swab sample from deep inside a man's nasal cavity with an arrow pointing to it with the words 'Implant microchip here'.

A whole crop of social media posts also started circulating in Arabic with millions of views, one with Gates photoshopped to look like The Joker with a white face and green hair and holding a giant needle. A Facebook page with a reference to a 'Horror Plan' by Gates to depopulate the planet racked up over 134,000 likes. As quickly as Facebook took down posts citing misinformation, more were springing up in every language. The monster that Gates helped create was now spawning unrelenting online attacks on the creator.

No matter that Gates had nothing to do with the drafting of H.R.6666 and was insistent he had no interest in tracking you to Tesco or the local Nando's, he was still getting the blame. And when he denied any knowledge, the conspiracy theorists came back with the old refrain, 'Well he would say that, wouldn't he?'

CHAPTER 16:

THE GREAT RESET
– 3 June 2020

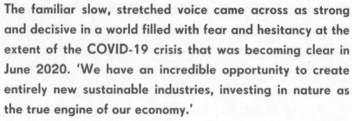

**The familiar slow, stretched voice came across as strong
and decisive in a world filled with fear and hesitancy at the
extent of the COVID-19 crisis that was becoming clear in
June 2020. 'We have an incredible opportunity to create
entirely new sustainable industries, investing in nature as
the true engine of our economy.'**

Panoramic scenes of melting ice floes, a stranded killer
whale, African villagers, green forests, giant dams, solar plants,
a kangaroo caught in wildfires and an empty Times Square flash
across the screen as he talks with the words:

RE-IMAGINE

RE-THINK

RE-INVENT

RE-DESIGN

RE-VIVE

RE-CREATE

RE-FORM

RE-BALANCE

RE-VOLUTION

And finally ... RE-SET

It is a call to action. The voice with its earnest cut-glass tone telling the world that it is time to rip up the rule books and start again.

'Changing our current trajectory will require bold and imaginative action together with determination and decisive leadership,' he continues. 'In order to secure our future and to prosper we need to evolve our economic model putting people and planets at the heart of global value creation. If there is one critical lesson we have to learn from this crisis; we need to put nature at the heart of how we operate. We are on the verge of catalytic breakthroughs that will alter our views of what is possible and profitable within the framework of a sustainable future. We need nothing short of a paradigm shift, one that inspires action at revolutionary levels and pace. We simply cannot waste any more time. The only limit is our willingness to act. And the time to act is now.'

So, who is this man calling for a revolution in the midst of one of the planet's worst pandemics? Read the words without hearing the voice and he could be a fringe extremist hell-bent on change with a bold vision and a poor sense of timing.

But this is Prince Charles, heir to the crown, and his video was released to great fanfare on 3 June 2020, on the Royal Family's YouTube channel. A sincere man who was way ahead of his time on climate change, Charles undoubtedly saw the COVID-19 outbreak as a catalyst for change and from his lockdown isolation in the grand halls of Buckingham Palace or from the perfectly manicured wild gardens of his Highgrove estate in the Cotswolds he clearly thought the world was prepped and ready for a green revolution.

He wasn't alone. Klaus Schwab and his super-wealthy cronies in the World Economic Forum were on board, as well, and jumped on the prince's initiative as the theme for their annual billionaire's bash. The idea that it may be tone deaf didn't seem to register with the super-rich, many of whom had seen their profits soar during the pandemic. According to the *Washington Post*, the wealth of America's top nine titans – all involved in tech – shot up by more than $360 billion while COVID wreaked havoc on the lives of ordinary people.

Between 5 March 2020 and 5 March 2021, tech billionaires saw their net worth rise by:

Elon Musk (Tesla) – $118 billion

Jeff Bezos (Amazon) – $58 billion

Larry Page (Alphabet – Google's parent company) – $33 billion

Sergey Brin (Alphabet) – $32 billion

Mark Zuckerberg (Facebook) – $29 billion

Larry Ellison (Oracle) – $28 billion

Bill Gates (ex-Microsoft) – $24 billion

Steve Ballmer (ex-Microsoft) – $23 billion

Michael Dell (Dell Technologies) – $18 billion

(Source: Bloomberg Billionaires Index)

Streets were empty, families were kept apart from their loved ones, businesses were failing and floundering, health workers were overwrought and overworked, babies were being born in isolation and grandparents were dying alone. And the 1 per cent was getting richer and richer.

'While millions are out of work and being evicted, the billionaire class thrived and prospered as they seldom have in any year,' Anand Giridharadas, author of *Winners Take All: The Elite Charade of Changing the World*, told the *Washington Post*.

Ironically, Bill Gates, who gave away more of his personal

wealth ($1.75 billion) than any of his rival tech titans, took the most flak from conspiracy theorists. But Prince Charles and the super-wealthy elite who signed on to his campaign for a 'Global Reset' were about to find themselves in the firing line of critics who either saw it as an idealistic dream that would only serve to hand over more power to the rich and powerful – or a cunning culling plot by the elite to take over the world.

Few people were prepared to believe that the very people who benefited the most from the pandemic were willing to forgo the capitalistic system that made them world leaders and multi-billionaires in favour of a more benevolent, fairer society. Would they give up greed for good? Spread the wealth? No, didn't think so.

However well intentioned, Prince Charles' attempt to boost interest in his sustainable reset may have got little traction outside royal watchers and his loyal friends who have long been irritated by his public image as a frustrated David Attenborough who talks to his plants.

But earlier in 2020, the World Economic Forum's decision to try a sustainable theme for its 2020 Davos summit in the Swiss Alps gave Charles a higher international profile and offered him a major platform to expand on his idea. Guests at the fiftieth anniversary event ranged from Donald Trump to Greta Thunberg. Still unaware of the toll in lives and lifestyle that the pandemic was about to unleash, the world's most exclusive club gathered in person at the mountain hideaway to pay lip service, at the least, to the annual meeting's tagline, 'Stakeholders for a Cohesive and Sustainable World'.

Introducing the prince, Schwab, the German economist behind the WEF, said Charles' decision to return to the summit stage after thirty years was because the world was reaching a 'global tipping point' in areas 'so close to the heart of His Royal Highness'.

Charles started his speech talking about being 'in the midst of a crisis that is now, I hope, well understood'. He wasn't referring to COVID. We still don't really understand that one and, at that point, the Chinese were still trying desperately to keep it contained. 'Global warming, climate change and the devastating loss of biodiversity are the greatest threats humanity has ever faced and one largely of our own creation,' Charles continued.

'Now I have dedicated much of my life to the restoration of harmony between humanity, nature and the environment and to the encouragement of corporate, social and environmental responsibility. Quite frankly, it has been a bit of an uphill struggle, but now it is time to take it to the next level,' he added.

It is at this point that the prince starts his pitch to his well-heeled audience. 'In order to secure our future and to prosper, we need to evolve our economic model. Having been engaged in these issues since 1968 when I made my first speech on the environment and having talked to countless experts across the globe over those decades, I have come to realise that it is not a lack of capital that is holding us back but rather the way in which we deploy it. Therefore, to move forward, we need nothing short of a paradigm shift, one that requires action at revolutionary levels and pace. With this in mind, I am delighted to be launching a sustainable markets initiative with the generous support of the World Economic Forum.'

The prince went on to list ten ways he wanted the business and government leaders present to boost sustainability, ideas such as investing in nature, in research and development and ticking off businessmen who have previously put profit over climate change. Coming to a close, he promised to set up round tables 'bringing together system innovators and decision makers to start designing and charting the course'.

'I believe profoundly in the critical importance of this juncture of forming an unprecedented global alliance of investors, which can genuinely mobilise the kind of trillions of dollars needed to put our economy on the correct path. This would be the most dramatic act of responsible leadership ever seen by the global private sector and would at once provide a catalytic incentive for the public sector to follow.

'So, with 2020 being seen as the super year kick-starting a decade of action for people and planet, there is also an opportunity to bring sustainable markets into focus in each of this year's major global meetings, while it will be a bit of a challenge for me to get to them all. I tend to do my utmost to ensure that the message of urgent systemic change, collaboration and integration is heard.

'After all, ladies and gentlemen, do we want to go down in history as the people who did nothing to bring the world back from the brink in time to restore the balance when we could have done? I don't want to and just think for a moment, what good is all the extra wealth in the world gained from business as usual if you could do nothing with it, except watch it burn in catastrophic conditions? This is why I need your help, your ingenuity and your practical skills to ensure that the private sector leads the world out of the approaching catastrophe into which we have engineered ourselves.

'It is my greatest possible hope that you will join me this year in accelerating the transition to sustainable markets and rapid decarbonisation. Ladies and gentlemen, you all have a seat at the table as this must be the year that we put ourselves on the right track. Everything I've tried to do and urge over the past fifty years has been done with our children and grandchildren in mind, because I did not want to be accused by them of doing nothing except prevaricate and deny the problem.

'Now, of course, they are accusing us of exactly that. So put yourselves in their position, ladies and gentlemen, we simply cannot waste any more time. The only limit, the only limit is our willingness to act. And the time to act is now.'

Now this may not sound like a call for a revolution, although, in a sense that is what the prince was asking for. The topic went down well enough for 'The Great Reset' to be adopted as the title slogan for the 2021 Davos summit when, presumably, the prince hoped to press home his message.

Then came the pandemic and Charles was among the first famous people to test positive in March 2020, complaining of mild symptoms and banishing himself to the queen's Scottish estate at Balmoral for seven days (he also caught COVID in February 2022).

By June, the prince was ready with the cooperation of Schwab to launch his Great Reset with his shiny YouTube video and a publicity push aided by the WEF. In an interview, Charles doubled down on his earlier statements in spite of the ravages of the pandemic, saying: 'We have a unique but rapidly shrinking window of opportunity to learn lessons and reset ourselves on a more sustainable path. It is an opportunity we have never had before and may never have again so we must use all the levers we have at our disposal knowing that each and every one of us has a vital role to play.

'We have no alternative because otherwise, unless we take the action necessary and we build again in a greener, more sustainable and more inclusive way, then we will end up having more and more pandemics and more and more disasters from ever-accelerating global warming and climate change. This is the one moment, as you've all been saying, when we have to make as much progress as we can.'

On the Prince of Wales official web page, the launch was explained in a single paragraph: 'The Great Reset, which was launched during a virtual round table today, aims to rebuild, redesign, reinvigorate and rebalance our world. It has been designed to ensure businesses and communities 'build back better' by putting sustainable business practices at the heart of their operations as they begin to recover from the corona-virus pandemic.'

There was also a tweet from Prince Charles and The Duchess of Cornwall that read: '#TheGreatReset initiative is designed to ensure businesses and communities "build back better" by putting sustainable business practices at the heart of their operations as they begin to recover from the coronavirus pandemic.'

Schwab weighed in with a book – *The Great Reset: Resetting the World* – and an article timed for the June launch in which the founder and executive chairman of the WEF expanded on the idea that COVID had created an opportunity for change.

'One silver lining of the pandemic is that it has shown how quickly we can make radical changes to our lifestyles,' he wrote on the WEF website. 'Almost instantly, the crisis forced businesses and individuals to abandon practices long claimed to be essential, from frequent air travel to working in an office. Likewise, populations have overwhelmingly shown a willingness to make sacrifices for the sake of healthcare and other essential workers and vulnerable populations, such as the elderly. And many companies have stepped up to support their workers, customers and local communities, in a shift towards the kind of stakeholder capitalism to which they had previously paid lip service.

'Clearly,' continued Schwab, 'the will to build a better society does exist. We must use it to secure the Great Reset that we so badly need. That will require stronger and more effective governments, though this does not imply an ideological push for *bigger* ones. And it will demand private-sector engagement every step of the way...

'The COVID-19 crisis is affecting every facet of people's lives in every corner of the world. But tragedy need not be its only legacy,' he concludes. 'On the contrary, the pandemic represents a rare but narrow window of opportunity to reflect, reimagine, and reset our world to create a healthier, more equitable, and more prosperous future.'

Suddenly, the conspiracy theorists were in play.

The prince's vague plan to restructure the planet's economy to make it greener and more sustainable became an evil plot by the globalist elite to rule the world. Because it is more of a concept than a blueprint for change, the Great Reset is ripe for conspiracy theories to fill in the gaps, so much so that it has grown to become one of the pandemic's most popular and most widespread theories. This time we don't just have Bill Gates but a whole bunch of super-wealthy elites who supposedly share the ambitions of a James Bond villain.

According to a BBC investigation, the term The Great Reset had more than 8 million interactions on Facebook and was shared over 2 million times on Twitter in the year after Prince Charles' 3 June 2020 launch. There were 178,000 Facebook posts in total with the most popular posts 'baseless statements that the Great Reset is a strategic part of a grand conspiracy by the global elite, who somehow planned and managed the COVID-19 pandemic'.

The online narrative was not so much about a benevolent prince and his rich and powerful audience looking for a way to make the world a better place, but the idea that lockdowns were not to save lives but to control the populace and bring about an economic catastrophe that would give the elites the opening they needed to create a socialist cabal of world leaders. The irony of capitalists and a royal, to boot, apparently seeking a socialist revolution was not lost on sceptics.

One clue to the viral boom in posts linking the reset with socialism was in the use of the phrase 'build back better' on the Prince of Wales's web page. It was also the name of Democrat President Joe Biden's multi-billion dollar 'Build Back Better' plan that was strongly opposed by Republicans on Capitol Hill. It's unlikely that the prince was aware of the connection when the phrase was used, but it was jumped on by conservatives in America and was widely quoted as evidence of a left-wing plot.

Another spike in traction came in November 2020 when Canadian Prime Minister Justin Trudeau, speaking on a United Nations video conference, said he met with other leaders to discuss 'fundamental gaps and inequities' in the respective countries. He went on to say the 'pandemic provided an opportunity for a reset', and to 're-imagine economic systems'. Trudeau even used the words 'building back better'.

The BBC reported that 1.8 million tweets used the keywords or hashtag 'Great Reset' between June 2020 and May 2021 with the biggest spike of around 450,000 tweets when the UN video of Trudeau's remarks went viral.

Adopting the socialist takeover narrative, Trump supporters used it to claim that the former reality star's re-election to the White House was the only way to prevent the rich revolution.

That was certainly the message from a senior figure in the Catholic Church who stoked the speculation with a serious dose of fire and brimstone.

Archbishop Carlo Maria Viganò, a former secretary-general of the governorate of Vatican City State and Apostolic Nuncio to the US – the Vatican's 'ambassador' in Washington – had already courted controversy for some years by exposing corruption and sexual abuse in the church when he wrote an open letter to then President Trump on 25 October 2020, claiming the 'fate of the whole world is being threatened by a global conspiracy against God and humanity'.

Published in the *Catholic Family News*, the archbishop described the pandemic as 'the forces of Evil aligned in a battle without quarter against the forces of Good; forces of Evil that appear powerful and organized as they oppose the children of Light, who are disoriented and disorganized, abandoned by their temporal and spiritual leaders.'

He claimed that basic human values such as family, respect for life, freedom, and love of country were under attack while national and religious leaders were 'pandering to this suicide of Western culture and its Christian soul'. He added that people's fundamental rights were being denied 'in the name of a health emergency that is revealing itself more and more fully as instrumental to the establishment of an inhuman faceless tyranny.'

In his cross-hairs was the Great Reset. The archbishop insisted it was being promoted under the guise of the pandemic by a global elite that 'wants to subdue all of humanity, imposing coercive measures with which to drastically limit individual freedoms and those of entire populations.'

'Behind the world leaders who are the accomplices and executors of this infernal project, there are unscrupulous characters who finance the World Economic Forum and Event 201, promoting their agenda,' he added.

Once again, Bill Gates gets a mention as the archbishop claimed the purpose of the Great Reset is to create a 'health dictatorship.' He repeated the idea that the elites were seeking the 'renunciation of private property' and 'adherence to a program of vaccination against COVID-19 and COVID-21 promoted by Bill Gates with the collaboration of the main pharmaceutical groups.'

'The imposition of the vaccination will be accompanied by the requirement of a health passport and a digital ID, with the consequent contact tracing of the population of the entire world,' he continued. 'Those who do not accept these measures will be confined in detention camps or placed under house arrest, and all their assets will be confiscated.'

The archbishop set the date for activation of the Great Reset as the end of 2020 and the beginning of 2021 and suggested further lockdowns were planned to fester discontent and provoke an economic crisis.

Viganò defended his use of 'apocalyptic' language to describe what he saw as an enormous threat that was being executed under our noses with the complicity of the mainstream media. He also hit out at those smearing opponents of the Great Reset as 'conspiracy theorists,'

'No one, up until last February, would ever have thought that, in all of our cities, citizens would be arrested simply for wanting to walk down the street, to breathe, to want to keep their business open, to want to go to church on Sunday,' he wrote. 'Yet now it is happening all over the world, even in picture postcard Italy that many Americans consider to be a small enchanted country, with its ancient monuments, its churches, its charming cities, its characteristic villages. And while the politicians are barricaded inside their palaces promulgating decrees like Persian satraps, businesses are failing, shops are closing, and people are prevented from living, traveling, working, and praying.'

He continued: 'The disastrous psychological consequences of this operation are already being seen, beginning with the suicides of desperate entrepreneurs and of our children, segregated from friends and classmates, told to follow their classes while sitting at home alone in front of a computer.'

The archbishop clearly saw President Trump as a kindred spirit, addressing him directly: 'Mr. President, you have clearly stated that you want to defend the nation – One Nation under God, fundamental liberties, and non-negotiable values that are denied and fought against today. It is you, dear President, who are 'the one who opposes' the deep state, the final assault of the children of darkness.'

He went on to declare his interest in the impending 2020 presidential election, leaving no doubt where his loyalties were, calling Trump the 'final garrison against the world dictatorship' and lambasting his rival and the eventual victor Joe Biden as 'a person who is manipulated by the deep state, gravely compromised by scandals and corruption, who will do to the United States what Jorge Mario Bergoglio is doing to the Church, Prime Minister Conte to Italy, President Macron to France, Prime Minster Sanchez to Spain, and so on.'

He continued: 'The blackmailable nature of Joe Biden – just like that of the prelates of the Vatican's 'magic circle' – will expose him to be used unscrupulously, allowing illegitimate powers to interfere in both domestic politics as well as international balances. It is obvious that those who manipulate him already have someone worse than him ready, with whom they will replace him as soon as the opportunity arises.'

The archbishop wrote that the Great Reset, enabled by

lockdowns, was 'destined to fail' because 'the enemy has Satan on its side, he who only knows how to hate. But on our side, we have the Lord Almighty, the God of armies arrayed for battle, and the Most Holy Virgin, who will crush the head of the ancient Serpent.'

In conclusion, he underlined his support for Trump and his supporters, writing: 'Mr. President, you are well aware that, in this crucial hour, the United States of America is considered the defending wall against which the war declared by the advocates of globalism has been unleashed. Place your trust in the Lord, strengthened by the words of the Apostle Paul: 'I can do all things in Him who strengthens me' (Phil 4:13). To be an instrument of Divine Providence is a great responsibility, for which you will certainly receive all the graces of state that you need, since they are being fervently implored for you by the many people who support you with their prayers.'

The bleak picture painted by the archbishop quickly became a cornerstone of the Great Reset conspiracy theory. His letter is sprinkled with conspirator key words such as references to a 'Deep State' and a 'New World Order' and the obligatory mention of Bill Gates.

Not surprisingly, all manner of people jumped on board with the theory after this, using the Great Reset conspiracy theory as a means to push their own specific agendas from disenfranchisement to Nazism and anti-Semitism to Trumpism.

Some took the whole thing another leap forward, suggesting the elites were plotting to turn the rest of us into robots or 'cyborgs'.

In a YouTube video, popular conspiracy theorist Spiro Skouras insisted COVID was an engineered disaster and claimed the 'Great Reset' was all about replacing humans with robots controlled by the elite. 'This is not about saving the planet, this is not about equality, this is about control,' he says. 'Many of the jobs will be taken by robots so they will redefine work and what it means to work. They want to redefine what it means to be human and determine for you your role and your future of being essentially a transhumanist cyborg integrated into this new control grid.

'Right now, we are witnessing the controlled demolition of the current system of control, by design, in order to usher in this new transhumanist agenda, this new system of global governance, this new digitalised system of control where we will be unable to distinguish organic life from artificial. We won't even have access to our own thoughts, or we'll have access to them, but we won't even be able to control our own thoughts and emotions because they're going to do that for us because we're going to be tied into their grid system.'

Central banks and governments didn't want to be blamed for dismantling the economic system as we knew it, he says. 'The virus is here to take the fall,' he insists. 'The virus is the excuse to burn down this old system. Out of these ashes the new system will rise. These technocrats are deciding the future of humanity for us right now and, guess what, the future of humanity isn't human at all...'

Right-wing TV hosts in the United States, and on Rupert Murdoch's Fox News, in particular, saw the Great Reset as an excuse to pile in on new Democrat President Joe Biden. Fox anchor Laura Ingraham, speaking on her 13 November 2020 show shortly after Biden's election victory, claimed the 'global elites' were 'anti-democratic control freaks' who had a different idea of the new normal on the other side of the pandemic.

'Come on, you know, they hated that old normal,' she said. 'They want a new normal and they don't like that old normal where Americans just enjoyed their freedoms, the freedoms we often took for granted like the right to work, to run a business, to attend school, the right to travel and so on.'

She claimed Biden was in league with Prince Charles, Klaus Schwab and the WEF's Great Reset initiative. 'The fact is, all the signs point to Joe Biden's team being fully on board with this cynical and sick perversion of American independence sovereignty,' she said, adding that he was using 'the fear of COVID hanging over our heads' to hand over veto power to Schwab and his elites.

'Bill Gates, the WHO, the World Economic Forum, Prince Charles, the IMF, big business and big tech, they're all in big for the Great Reset. If it means you have to give up your individual rights for global health security, so be it. Remember, surveillance, tracking, it's all good for you.'

Three days later, Tucker Carlson, another ultra-conservative Fox News anchor, was also taking aim at the Great Reset, pouring more oil on the conspiracy theories fires. He highlights the open letter written by 'truth teller' Catholic Archbishop Carlo Maria Viganò and asks: 'What does the Great Reset look like? This is what it looks like: The people in charge doing whatever they want because they're in charge. There will be no live music in the Great Reset. Choirs will be illegal unless they are singing the praises of Kamala Harris. Christmas will be banned. "Sorry, put on your mask and spend the holidays alone. Good luck."'

Fox News is not hidden away in a corner of the internet; it has been America's top-rated news network for the past twenty years and commands about half of the nation's entire cable news audience. These commentators are giving credibility to these views by the very nature of the kind of exposure they can give them.

On 16 December 2020, Glenn Beck, a former Fox host, called

COVID 'the gateway drug to global socialism – the Great Reset ... Capitalism itself is under attack and will change unless you stand up ... how you live your life is about to change and most people don't know.'

He claimed that John Kerry, then US Secretary of State, told the WEF that Biden 'will accelerate the great reset with greater intensity than people are expecting'. He added: 'Before I'm called a conspiracy theorist, these are his words, not mine.'

Even further down the conspiracy rabbit hole, Alex Jones, the rabid Infowars host, devoted a show to the subject called 'The Great Reset's End Game is Total Extermination of All Humans on Earth.' Pretty sure that's not what Prince Charles meant when he talked about changing the world for the better.

But then, the WEF wasn't exactly helping itself. On 18 November 2016, it posted a video with '8 predictions for the world in 2030' and number one showed a photo of a smiling, bearded man with the caption, 'You will own nothing, and you'll be happy.' It didn't take much researching for people worried about the implications of the Great Reset to find the video and draw their own conclusions.

'The purpose of this sleight of hand is to eliminate private property and small businesses (COVID?), which is the fundamental principle of prosperity. Funny! I will not own anything but I will have to rent ... which means that someone else will be the owner instead of me. Let me guess who! We are not stupids,' read one post.

'I'll be so happy when I own nothing and am forced to eat genetically modified tofu every day 😂 thanks Bill and friends at the WEF for planning to control my life ... god knows I couldn't make my own decisions for much longer ... such a burden choice is #thisiswhybidenwon,' read another. And there were plenty more.

To claims that the WEF's Great Reset concept of, 'You will own nothing, and you'll be happy' is a conspiracy theory even Russell Brand, the antithesis of the Fox News ranters, takes issue with. 'It's not really a conspiracy theory, is it?' he says on his YouTube channel. 'There's a video saying it and stuff. They've gone to a lot of trouble to make it look all nice.'

Brand highlights a purported 'land grab' by big investors paying over the top prices for family homes in the US to push out middle-class homeowners – an offshoot of the Great Reset theory that feeds into the 'own nothing' concept. 'We are talking about the movement of huge amounts of finance and speculating as to what the impact might be on ordinary people,' he says in a January 2022 video with more than two million views. 'Sometimes these things are dense and quite difficult to understand, and I think that's deliberate,' he adds, 'We have an obligation to personally investigate and make ourselves aware of what's happening because otherwise, you'll go, "Oh, that's a conspiracy theory," and dismiss it. No, this is what underwrites things that would otherwise be regarded as conspiracy theories. You can say something like, "You'll own nothing, and you'll be happy," and you'll think, "Piss off, don't tell me what to do," but somewhere don't you think, how are they going to do that? What are the phases going to be where property is extracted, where the ability to control your own resources is extracted? Well, it's this, centralized investment facilities will start to acquire resources that previously were the domain ... of single families. That's cultural engineering. That's using the interests of the powerful to alter an entire society.'

The WEF 'own nothing' video goes on to claim that by 2030, 'Whatever you want you'll rent and it will be delivered by drone, the US won't be the world leading superpower, a handful of countries will dominate...'

The Facebook post links to a story on the WEF forum website that offers a stark explanation of the 'own nothing' concept. It reads: 'I don't own anything. I don't own a car. I don't own a house. I don't own any appliances or any clothes,' writes Danish MP Ida Auken. Shopping is a distant memory in the city of 2030, whose inhabitants have cracked clean energy and borrow what they need on demand. It sounds utopian, until she mentions that her every move is tracked and outside the city live swathes of discontents, the ultimate depiction of a society split in two.

Whether you believe in Prince Charles' greener vision of the future or mistrust his motives and those of his powerful partners, the WEF seems to have made a right mess of the message. You would never describe it as a humble organisation, but even the WEF had to put its hands up and admit it made the Great Reset sound like a conspiracy theory.

In a 25 January 2021 video watched by more than 1.6 million people, the WEF doubled down on its stance that COVID provides a unique opportunity for change, while confessing a better presentation would have helped.

'With everything falling apart, we can reshape the world in ways we couldn't before, ways that better address so many of the challenges we face, and that's why so many are calling for a Great Reset,' a smooth-voiced narrator says over glossy scenes of world leaders, ordinary people and emotive landscapes.

But in a sudden change of tone, the voice asks: 'A Great Reset? That sounds more like Buzzword Bingo, masking some nefarious plan for world domination!' A silver hand appears on the screen manipulating a world on puppet strings in space. The backdrop is then dominated by a fake newspaper, the DAILY NEWS, with a story under the headline GLOBAL ELITE'S PLAN FOR YOUR FUTURE and sub-head THE GREAT RESET IS WELL

DOCUMENTED that reads: 'The Great Reset has been labelled a conspiracy theory and parts of it sound like a conspiracy theory, but everything we know about it comes from the global elites themselves, who have been quite open about it.'

The story is an apparent lift from an article by Dale Hurd on the Christian Broadcasting Network (CBN). It continues:

'This is not a conspiracy theory, this is a well-documented movement among many of the world's most powerful people,' says Justin Haskins, the editorial director at the Heartland Institute and a leading authority on the Great Reset. 'Fundamentally, this is a radical and complete transformation of everything that we do in our society,' Haskins adds, 'It will change the way businesses are evaluated, it will coerce businesses to pursue left-wing causes.' The Great Reset was unveiled at the World Economic Forum in Davos, Switzerland, where many of the world's most powerful people go to offer solutions to the world's problems. They have said that the coronavirus pandemic is a historic opportunity to change the way the world operates. *COVID-19 Pandemic as an 'Opportunity' to Change Everything.*

'A World Economic Forum video warns, "Right now we're facing a crisis of international proportions. It's going to have a long-term impact on us."

And their solution is essentially global socialism. Think of the Green New Deal combined with the COVID-19 lockdown restrictions and throw in something called the Fourth Industrial Revolution, in which technology is supposed to radically change the way we live and work.

Klaus Schwab, the founder of the World Economic Forum, says the Fourth Industrial Revolution will lead to '...a fusion of our physical, our digital and our biological identities'.

It has the support not only of world leaders but of global

corporations like Mastercard and BP and is brought to you by people who think they know what's best for you.

Haskins says: 'The elites, the technocrats in society, the most educated people,' see the chance to 'control and manipulate society, pull the levers in society so that it's in their minds, perfect'.

'*Standing in the Way: A Trump Re-election*

'But a Trump re-election would blow a massive hole in the Great Reset. One week before the election, Italian Archbishop Carlo Maria Viganò wrote an open letter to the President, warning him that the Great Reset is 'inhuman faceless tyranny' that seeks to 'subdue all of humanity', and that President Trump and the United States are the wall against 'the deep state, the final assault of the children of darkness'.

'Over the past four years, Donald Trump has been the single greatest roadblock for people who are pushing this internationalist globalist sort of agenda,' Haskins says.

The Elites' New Slogan: Build Back Better

The elites at Davos are now counting on a Biden victory for The Great Reset to go forward. The World Economic Forum and the Biden campaign even share the same slogan, 'Build back better'.

The mocked-up newspaper front page then gives way on screen to another fake front page, this time for THE DAILY HERALD with the headline 'HANDS UP'.

The story reads: 'Does building back better mean a "Great Reset", the end of our freedoms, and the dawn of global technocratic state? Many conspiracy theorists are beginning to think so.'

'Hands up,' says the narrator's voiceover, 'this kind of slogan hasn't gone down well, but all we really want to say is that we all have an opportunity to build a better world. And it's not surprising that people who have been disenfranchised by a broken system and pushed even further by the pandemic will suspect global leaders of conspiracy.

'But the world's not that simple,' it continues. 'Every one of us has differing priorities, values and ideas. That's part of why solutions are so hard to come by and why we all need to be involved in the decision making because whether it's politicians, CEOs, academics, activists, or you, we are all about getting people together, even those you may not like.'

A collage of world figures appears on the video, including Joe Biden, George Bush, Greta Thunberg, Ivanka Trump, Angela Merkel, David Attenborough ... and Vladimir Putin.

The video goes on to point out that at the outset of the pandemic at the beginning of 2020, 1 per cent of the world's population owned 44 per cent of its wealth. 'Since the start of the pandemic, billionaires have increased theirs by more than 25 per cent whilst 150 million people fell back into extreme poverty' and urges ordinary people to 'tune in, turn on and get involved' by following the DAVOS agenda.

So, can you have a conspiracy theory about something nobody is really trying to hide? Disregarding the more extreme theories, I don't see anyone at Davos suggesting the use of cyborgs or mass executions; the answer revolves around motive. Is there really a genuine feeling among the world's richest and most powerful minority to make the planet a better place for the rest of us? Do they really want a fairer distribution of wealth?

The evidence seems to suggest otherwise. If we have nothing and we're happy then who does own everything? And why would that make us happy?

Barack Obama's chief-of-staff Rahm Emanuel quipped during the 2008 financial crisis that, 'you never want a serious crisis to go to waste' and that seems to be what Charles and the WEF are saying now.

But the truth is that the rich often get richer during a crisis and, as we have seen, the COVID-19 pandemic was no exception.

As I have said, Charles may be a thoughtful, sensitive man living, as he does, in his ivory towers, but there is little evidence that the Great Reset is anything more than hollow words. The tech titans used their extra billions to toy with space travel; our political leaders enjoyed the kind of privileges they denied to others (Xmas party at Number 10, anyone?) and squabbling to the brink of World War III, and somehow, inexplicably, Wall Street profits kept rising – America's biggest bank, JPMorgan Chase made a $50 billion profit in 2021, about 35 per cent more than the $36 billion the bank made in 2019, the year before the pandemic. Goldman Sachs also announced record post-tax profits of $21.6 billion for 2021.

The money markets proved to be a COVID bonanza for the rich. While the rest of us were clapping our hands for the NHS every Thursday evening, the wealthy were rubbing their hands together.

Because the distribution of wealth has become so unequal, the revved-up markets didn't leave a mark on most middle-class households. In the United States in the third quarter of 2021, according to figures from the Federal Reserve quoted by *The New Yorker*, the top 1 per cent of households owned $21.6 trillion of stocks, the next wealthiest 9 per cent owned $14.1 trillion and the bottom 50 per cent, or half the country, owned just $300 billion.

Perhaps it's no wonder people get so suspicious when the rich and powerful suggest the rest of us should be happy not to own anything at all.

CHAPTER 17:

A FAMILY TORN APART BY COVID CONSPIRACY THEORIES
– 24 July 2021

With her coiffed blonde hair and glamorous outfits, Kate Shemirani became the poster woman for the anti-vaxxer movement with views so extreme that even notorious British conspiracy theorists like David Icke and Piers Corbyn distanced themselves from her.

She was struck off as a nurse, condemned for comparing efforts to control the spread of COVID to the Holocaust and insisted there was no evidence that there was a pandemic. Facebook, YouTube and Twitter all banned her for spreading misinformation.

Shemirani, a mother of four from East Sussex, was unrepentant. The more attention she received in the media, the more repugnant and more hectoring her statements became. On Twitter in September 2020, she asked when the public would wake up to what was happening: 'On the cattle truck? Or in the showers?'

Speaking at an anti-lockdown protest in Hyde Park, London in

July 2021, Shemirani, who had previously described the National Health Service as the 'new Auschwitz', urged the crowd to send her contact details for health workers, saying: 'Get their names. Email them to me. With a group of lawyers, we are collecting all that. At the Nuremberg Trials the doctors and nurses stood trial and they hung.'

When she was suspended for eighteen months by the Nursing and Midwifery Council over her coronavirus comments she said, according to *The Times*, that other nurses who complained about her were jealous and overweight. 'We all know what women can be like,' she said. 'The fact that I was always graced with decent looks and I'm always very slim and I've been very successful has generated a little bit of jealousy throughout my career.'

Her extreme views – calling the outbreak a 'scamdemic' and a 'plandemic' and an excuse for governments to control people's minds – have not only put her in contention with the authorities. They have also put her at odds with her own family.

In that, Shemirani is far from alone. In homes around the world, differing beliefs about the causes of the pandemic and the means of controlling it have caused rifts, some of them unassailable, between family members. In the most serious cases, belief in misinformation has led to deaths. Arguments over the merits of vaccination, wearing a mask and, yes, in some cases whether there was a pandemic at all, have wrecked countless families and friendships.

Shemirani's son revealed in an interview with the BBC how his family has paid a price for her emergence as a notorious conspiracy theorist. At the time, Sebastian Shemirani was twenty-one and studying at the London School of Economics and said he felt compelled to come forward to warn the public about his 'dangerous' mother.

'Thousands of people are taking her to be this source of truth and this saint, and I wish I could tell them all my mum is not the person that you think she is,' he explained. 'She's someone with a massive amount of self-interest and loves being at the centre of attention.'

He told how the family realised their issues with their mother had suddenly become a much bigger issue. 'My brother rings me,' he said, 'and he says, "Sebastian, I think we've got a problem – mum's got 40,000 YouTube followers." At that point my face just dropped. I knew immediately what was going on. This is her five minutes of fame. I don't want to be here talking about, you know, but I think it's something that we have got to do before these ideas get bigger and more people fall down the same route that she's trying to take them down. You can only prevent it before it happens.'

He was shocked to see a far-right contingent at his mother's rallies. 'My dad's Iranian and all of her kids are mixed race and she's out there getting all this clout and attention from people who don't think I should exist and definitely wouldn't like to listen to her if they did any digging whatsoever,' he said.

Asked what it was like growing up with Shemirani as his mother, Sebastian replied: 'The short answer is that it was hell. It's difficult to explain because we didn't live in particularly economically difficult circumstances. We had a nice big house in a good town.' But he said his mother would 'start playing these YouTube videos for me about how the Rothschilds are plotting to go live on a space station and how there's going to be this mass genocide, stuff like that. I'm ten, eleven years old and I'm bricking it, you know, I can't believe that the genocide is coming.'

Sebastian said he left home at seventeen. 'She came to see me as part of the global plot. She sent me a text a couple of weeks ago, saying, 'You need to listen to me. If you don't, you and your sister are going to die. The CIA has a plot. Half the UK's population is going to be killed within five years.'

'So, I asked who is going to benefit from this? No response, the rant continues. I think she's too far gone to be helped. I'm never going to have a relationship with my mum again. And that's why it's important that if someone else is coming to you and saying, "I'm starting to believe this stuff" – nip it in the bud because it takes a couple of years to completely lose somebody.

'And when this is over in three or four years' time, and everything she's said is forgotten, and the global genocide hasn't happened, people will forget about it. But the disaster that goes on within my family and the relationships that she's losing now, that stuff stays for ever.'

Shemirani's only response to the interview was to tell the BBC: 'From what I can see it would appear that a conspiracy theorist is actually now anyone who believes something other than what your controllers want them to believe. I find this deeply disturbing.'

The postman's daughter from Nottingham was a registered nurse for thirty-five years before she was struck off. She was reportedly diagnosed with breast cancer in 2012 but refused chemotherapy after undergoing a double mastectomy and has since followed a strict alternative medicine fat-free, salt-free, sugar-free vegan regime.

In the Nursing and Midwifery Council record of the hearing on misconduct charges brought against Shemirani, held between 26 and 28 May 2021, at the organisation's headquarters in Montfichet Road, London, it was said that the NMC received a 'significant' number of complaints about the state registered nurse.

'The Registrant has become a leading activist, speaker and promoter against vaccines and the existence of COVID-19,' it says about Shemirani. 'The Registrant has propagated the view that there is not currently a global COVID-19 pandemic, and that members of the nursing profession and other healthcare professionals are complicit in genocide.

'The Registrant has also encouraged the public not to follow advice from healthcare professionals, the medical community, the WHO and UK Government including on how to respond to and treat ill health caused by COVID-19, the flu and measles,' it continues. 'She has done this by way of social media, the internet, radio and TV interviews and at public events, including at a large protest in Trafalgar Square in London. The Registrant is a prolific user of social media. Her social media brand appears to be "Kate Shemirani – Natural Nurse in a Toxic World". At the time of the initial referrals the Registrant was active on multiple social media sites including Facebook, Twitter, YouTube and Instagram ... The Registrant's social media accounts have had a significant following. The Registrant's own claim is that collectively the videos and comments she posts to her social media platforms have been viewed over a million times. The Registrant has also stated that she had approximately 100,000 Facebook followers and that a video she recorded and posted to Facebook and Instagram had been viewed over 1 million times. The schedule of media files produced indicates that the Registrant's videos, posts and social media appearances usually reach in excess of 3,000 people, with some videos having up to 40,000 views at the time of recording...

'The Registrant's social media accounts with Facebook, Twitter, YouTube and Instagram have since been blocked by the respective organisations. The Registrant has however continued to post similar content and feature on other persons' accounts regularly on other social media sites such as Telegram, BitChute and Brighteon.

A report of the hearing outlines some of Shemirani's claims and her comments. It reads:

> The Registrant's comments and advice given in respect of the COVID-19 pandemic and vaccines include, although are not limited to, the following:
>
> a. denies that there is a global COVID-19 pandemic.
>
> b. states that 'there is no evidence that a pandemic exists, no evidence that Sars/COVID-2 has been purified and is unequivocally in existence'.
>
> c. states that vaccines have been 'rushed through' because 'they want to kill you'.
>
> d. states that 'I am a nurse. I don't agree with the vaccines anymore because I know what's in them.'
>
> e. attributes the symptoms of COVID-19 to radiation from 5G technology.
>
> f. describes the pandemic as a scam.
>
> g. states that 'you can't catch a virus.'
>
> h. describes vaccines as poison.
>
> i. states the flu vaccine causes long-term health issues that can be fatal and causes damage to brain cells, vital organs and dementia.
>
> j. states that vaccines cause sterility and changes a person's DNA.
>
> k. states that the ingredients in vaccines include acetone and aborted foetal cell tissue that turns into cancer.

l. advocates that members of the public and their children should not agree to be vaccinated against flu or measles.

m. states that no vaccine has ever been proved safe and effective.

n. suggested that ingesting disinfectant is less harmful than the ingredients of vaccines.

o. suggests that HPV vaccines cause cancer, had 'killed girls on the spot' and had led to death.

p. encouraged members of the public not to socially distance but to 'get hugging'.

q. discourages members of the public from wearing masks, stating that they do not stop viruses.

r. states that wearing a mask makes people very sick and increases the risk of bacteria and the risk of infections.

s. states that a person ill with COVID-19 may help other people by coughing on them.

The Registrant has also spoken and posted comments about nurses, other healthcare professionals, the NHS and the NMC. The comments made by the Registrant include, although is not limited to, the following:

a. that nurses and other healthcare professionals are currently murdering patients.

b. describe nurses as being complicit in murder and are criminals and liars.

c. compare nurses in the UK today with healthcare professionals who cooperated in the Nazi extermination and euthanasia programmes of the 1930s and 1940s.

d. describe healthcare professionals and vaccination teams as needing to be renamed death squads.

e. suggest that the National Institute for Clinical

Excellence ('NICE') has given healthcare professionals a 'licence to kill'.

    f. suggest that 9 out of every 10 nurses are 'crap'.

    g. describe nurses as being complicit in genocide.

    h.state that 'lots of nurses are really shit'.

    i. describe the NHS as 'murdering patients', 'genocidal', having been subject to 'Nazification'.

    j. state that hospitals practise 'bullshit medicine'.

    k. describe 'our elderly being systematically culled'.

    l. describe the NMC being 'lying liars of lies', 'complicit in murder', 'corrupt' and 'complicit in genocide'.

    m. describe the NMC as working to facilitate an agenda to 'cancel life-saving treatments in order to cause premature death', 'murder the old, infirm, disabled, vulnerable and sick', 'deceive and coerce the public to follow the lying government COVID agenda' and to 'support the racqueterring [*sic*] of the NHS'.

    n. state that the NHS, the NMC, the GMC, Public Health England and the Government are liars and conspiracy theorists, and should not be trusted.

    o. call for nurses and doctors as well as the Government to be arrested.

Backing the NMC's accusation that Shemirani was inflammatory and/or derogatory in her language, the disciplinary panel noted a number of examples, including the following: 'Without the help of the Doctors and Nurses, the extermination of Jews, gypsies, homosexuals, blacks, disabled... in the Holocaust could not have been executed...'[*sic*].

'Can I state the obvious. There is no COVID19. It's a scam. There is however contaminated vaccines, contaminated tests and a lovely direct energy weapon system being primed to activate those nano particles you have injected, ingested and inhaled'[sic].

'You health care professionals... I use that term lightly... infact... The Nurse vaccination teams need to be renamed DEATH SQUADS!'[sic].

'You are not nurses. You are not angels. You are criminals and liars'. 'Your hero status is well gone. The NMC are corrupt and common purpose. I wear that [interim] suspension [order from the NMC] like a badge of honour. It doesn't effect my excellent work and reputation. Many of you are murdering patients. Or looking on...You are rapidly turning into Angels of death. Speak up now. Or remain complicit in a crime against humanity'[sic].

'For all those foolish COVIDiots out there thinking I am in any way concerned about not being on a corrupt organisations register. I am not. I am far above being associated with a Common Purpose organisation that has worked to facilitate an agenda to:

1) cancel life-saving treatments in order to cause premature death

2) murder the old, infirm, disabled, vulnerable and sick

3) Hide, deceive and coerce the public to follow the lying government COVID agenda.

4) support the RACQUETERRING of the NHS...the industry formerly known as the healthcare system, swindling donations, discounts, food parcels for staff on full pay when there are many far more deserving and in need. For those that danced in full uniform and PPE gear thinking you were funny or entertaining ... you were not. You are a disgrace. An embarrassment. You have damaged a flagging job that used to be a profession. Shame on each of you...The NMC is a corrupt organisation facilitating and covering up murder of patients within NHS and private facilities... Nurses have been given a 'license to kill' from NICE

on April 29th 2020, 'patients scoring 6 or above on the critical frailty score who cannot reach their desired goals, can have all treatment removed'. This is murder...'[*sic*].

'We are now in possession of enough evidence against the NMC in relation to the facilitation of the TERRORIST AGENDA TO COMMIT GENOCIDE'.

'Friend just sent me her txt! Pimps for pharma. The Nazification of the NHS formerly known as the health care industry'[*sic*].

'This is a conspiracy to commit mass Genocide and there is prima facie evidence to support this. Contaminated vaccines increase the lethality of 5G and the switch on in Wuhan confirmed the pathogens activation using microwave radiation as a weapon'[sic]

'Patients all with DNRs on arrival. Patient and relatives unaware. Murdered. Genocide. The NHS is the new Auschwitz. 4th generation warfare. Silent weapons for quiet wars. You are the target'.

'Unlawful "do not resuscitate" orders are being placed on patients with a learning disability during the coronavirus pandemic without families being consulted. I call it Genocide. Nurses and Drs of 'The Third Reich''[sic].

'This is called "Terrorism" against the children of the world. But we must remember that the WHO is indeed ran by Tedros The Terrorist [The director general of the WHO]'.

Stating why the NMC decided to strike off the renegade nurse, it explained:

Mrs Shemirani's misconduct was of the utmost serious-ness and was not a one-off incident. In the panel's view, she has embarked upon a calculated course of conduct, intending to cause distress, panic and alarm amongst the general population, as well as being offensive to the nursing and healthcare profession. Mrs Shemirani has used her platform to promote her own propaganda and encourage people to act contrary to public health guidance during the COVID-19 pandemic.

Sebastian later tweeted about his mother's anti-COVID campaigning after learning an old school friend had died from the virus. 'Today I learned that a childhood friend of mine, who my mum used to drive to school with me, has died of COVID complications while working as a junior doctor,' he wrote. 'She was one of the smartest and loveliest girls I ever knew. And my mum was campaigning to put her at risk. So angry.

'My mum is a conspiracy theorist who believes COVID is made up by the "global elite" and the vaccine will kill us all. As such she rejects all forms of social distancing and recommends we all act like COVID doesn't exist. I'd like us to act like she doesn't exist.'

He told his followers later that he had told his mother what happened. 'Update: I told my mum the news. She blames the vaccine, even though my friend died before the vaccine was rolled out,' he wrote.

When someone tweeted that he should forgive his mother, Sebastian replied: 'No, this isn't a case where forgiveness applies. Her role as a mother has long passed. Who knows how many people have died because of my mum's lies? To forgive her is up to God, to fight her in this life is up to us. I can't help thinking if I'd have argued harder/earlier then her impact would've been smaller. Feeling some kind of survivor guilt right now.'

Sebastian told BBC's Radio 4 that his mother should be

prosecuted. 'If there aren't existing laws in place that say that what she is doing is illegal then we should be having a national conversation about what laws we should be bringing in and drafting up legislation for that because it's only a matter of time before some react on the bad advice she is giving the country,' he said in an interview watched more than 425,000 times on Twitter.

'I wouldn't say that most people who believe these ideas are beyond it. It may take a few years, but you eventually cool down from an initial radical period and you start listening to people around you more. But my mum is definitely beyond help.

'The problem is that because she's so arrogant in her world view and really truly believes that she is a conduit for the truth, on a spiritual level not just a scientific level, that she's been anointed by God or some other higher power, she thinks she shouldn't have to listen to other people like us, and every time I have tried to argue with her, either in a nice, calm, rational way in which I ask her questions and try and get her own argument into knots, or if I just straight up disagree and say you're wrong, either way she will end up getting irate at me and saying that I'm arrogant and that I don't listen to her. So, it's impossible to talk to somebody when they've got that level of God complex.'

Whatever you may think of Shemirani, and she is nothing if not consistent in her tirades against the way the British authorities have handled a pandemic she somehow believes to be a hoax, she has paid a price for her beliefs. She was struck off as a nurse, investigated by the police for her inflammatory remarks, banned from Facebook, YouTube and Twitter and, it seems, has lost some members of her family.

It is interesting to compare her fate with another outspoken blonde who shares many of the same beliefs but lives in the United States.

Marjorie Taylor Greene has also been a steadfast opponent of face masks during the pandemic, comparing mandates to the treatment of Jews during the Holocaust, and refused to get a vaccine because she was 'perfectly healthy'. She has been linked with the QAnon movement, although she now denies any connection, stories about her online are among the most read, a fact borne out by page views on mainstream sites detailing her remarks, and she has toured the US riling up rally crowds with her anti-vaxxer rhetoric. She also has a history as a conspiracy theorist, falsely claiming that 9/11 was a hoax, insisting that Barack Obama was a Muslim and accusing the Clintons of murder. According to the *New York Times*, she once claimed that a California wildfire was started by a 'laser' beam from space controlled by a Jewish banking family and reportedly went on social media to 'like' a Facebook comment suggesting 'a bullet to the head' to remove Democrat House Speaker Nancy Pelosi.

What became of Greene? She was elected to US Congress in November 2020, as the first woman representing Georgia's 14th District and Donald Trump acclaimed her as a rising star of the Republican Party.

Britain denounces Shemirani while the US embraces MTG. Much of the reason for that disparity is America's politicisation of the pandemic. Greene was stripped from membership of committees in the House of Representatives and reprimanded over twenty times by the House Serjeant-at-Arms and fined a total of more than $48,000 for refusing to wear a mask in the chamber of the Capitol, and Democrats routinely rubbished her as a far-right rabble-rouser. But much in the way that dyed-in-the-wool Republicans put up with Trump because of his enormous popularity in the country, party leaders were reticent about admonishing Greene because voters seemed to be on board with her conspiratorial theories.

Greene came out all guns blazing when questioned about her beliefs, tweeting in January 2021 that she was being targeted by the 'radical, left-wing Democrat mob' and claiming: 'If Republicans cower to the mob, and let the Democrats and the fake news media take me out they're opening the door to come after every single Republican until there's none left.' She supported the 'Stop the Steal' movement backing the baseless claim that Trump won the 2020 election and called the Republican candidate's removal from the White House 'an attack on every American who voted for him'.

Shemirani and Greene undoubtedly have their followers, many more than you might think. But only one of them numbers a former President of the United States among them.

They are also far from alone in comparing attempts to keep people safe in the pandemic, whether or not you agree with the methods, to Nazi Germany's despicable attempts to exterminate an entire ethnoreligious group.

The comparisons were not restricted to conspiracy theorists, either. Marcus Fysh, the Tory MP for Yeovil, likened the British government's planned COVID restrictions to the Nazis in an interview on BBC Radio 5 Live in December 2021 as he threatened to vote against Prime Minister Boris Johnson's latest round of measures. He appeared particularly angered over plans requiring proof of double vaccinations or a negative lateral flow test to be allowed into some events.

Fysh said he was opposed to 'segregating society based on an unacceptable thing', adding: 'We are not a "papers please" society. This is not Nazi Germany. It's the thin end of an authoritarian wedge and that's why we will resist it.'

His remarks led to an immediate backlash, with the Board of Deputies of British Jews saying: 'It is completely unacceptable to compare the proposed vaccine passports with Nazi Germany. We urge people, particularly those in positions of authority, to avoid these highly inappropriate comparisons.'

Deputy Prime Minister Dominic Raab, whose father was a Jewish refugee, admonished his Conservative colleague, telling the *Today* programme on Radio 4: 'I don't like that kind of language and I don't think it's appropriate. Actually, I don't think comparing what we are trying to achieve to an authoritarian or Nazi regime is quite right. I think a lot of people find that crass.'

Across the Atlantic on Capitol Hill, House Minority Leader Kevin McCarthy also took the rare move of standing up to Marjorie Taylor Greene after she twice used Nazi comparisons to COVID mandates, saying: 'Marjorie is wrong, and her intentional decision to compare the horrors of the Holocaust with wearing masks is appalling.'

Taylor Greene made amends by visiting the Holocaust Museum in Washington, but it didn't stop her from using the comparison again, this time using the phrase 'medical brown shirts' to describe vaccination attempts.

Lauren Boebert, another pro-Trump, pro-guns, far-right Republican voted into the House of Representatives in 2020, also called people promoting vaccinations 'needle Nazis' and, mirroring Fysh's comments in the UK, Congressman Madison Cawthorn said he thought the idea of vaccine passports 'smacks of 1940s Nazi Germany' and claimed: 'We must make every effort to keep America from becoming a "show your papers society".'

In response to a tweet that read, 'What's the difference between vaccine papers and a yellow star? 82 years,' Kelli Ward,

Chairwoman of the Arizona Republican Party, wrote: 'Exactly, #WakeUpAmerica.'

There are other examples of state lawmakers making similarly inappropriate and offensive comparisons. Such was the anger over the kind of remarks emanating from elected officials that the Dallas Holocaust and Human Rights Museum felt compelled to issue a statement saying: 'Some of those who oppose stay-at-home and shelter-in-place requirements have charged state officials with behaving like Hitler and imposing Nazi-style orders. One such accusation, made last week by an elected official in Idaho against that state's governor, compared him to Hitler noting that in Nazi Germany "non-essential workers got put on a train". For the record, Hitler and the Nazis put Jews on trains – men, women, and children – to their deaths, not because they were non-essential workers, but simply because they were Jewish. This accusation is as disgraceful as it is historically insupportable and morally reprehensible. The deportation of Jews to their deaths by a totalitarian, racist, antisemitic regime stands as an unmatched horrific time in modern history. To compare this to the efforts of our elected officials to attempt to balance our health and economic needs while under threat from a worldwide pandemic cheapens the sacrifice of the millions of Jews murdered by the Nazis and their collaborators.

'This statement is unacceptable and discouraging all the more because it was made by an elected official. More than ever, at a time when it is easy for fear and hate to take the place of compassion and kindness, we are committed to our mission to teach the history of the Holocaust and advance human rights to combat prejudice, hatred, and indifference. With antisemitism on the rise all over the world, we take this moment to choose acceptance, understanding, and respect. We hope you will join us today to remember, to hope, and to pledge: Never Again.'

Jewish leaders in New England said such remarks fuelled Holocaust deniers, quoting a study claiming that 23 per cent of respondents said, 'they believed the Holocaust was a myth, or had been exaggerated, or they were not sure.'

Nearly half (49 per cent) said they had seen Holocaust denial posts or distortions online.

'As Jewish leaders dedicated to advancing civil rights and public health, we are alarmed by the sharp rise of antisemitism in the criticism of COVID-19 mitigation measures,' wrote Robert Trestan, Executive Director of the Anti-Defamation League's New England office, and Becca Rausch, the first Jewish person to represent the Norfolk, Bristol and Middlesex District in the Massachusetts State Senate. 'Whether in public hearings, on social media or in the streets, we have heard far too many vaccine and mask opponents equate the policies keeping our communities safe to Nazi Germany. Rejecting public health practices is dangerous; weaponizing the Holocaust to attack these policies is both historically inaccurate and beyond unconscionable. The genocide of over eleven million people is incomparable to the measures necessary to combat a global pandemic,' they added.

'When COVID deniers and people who refute data-driven public health policy wrongly invoke the Holocaust, they pervert history, trivialize the memories of victims and survivors, and desensitize people to the monstrous atrocities that occurred,' they continued and gave several examples involving local politicians in the November 2021 article.

'Amidst historic levels of antisemitism and record reports of hate crimes,' they wrote, 'many leaders have exploited the horrors of the Holocaust for the sake of a sound bite. In August,

Maine Rep. Heidi Sampson, speaking at a rally protesting vaccine mandates for healthcare workers, compared Maine Gov. Janet Mills to Josef Mengele, the infamous Nazi doctor who conducted heinous 'experiments' on Jews and other Nazi prisoners. When she asked the crowd to recall 'the '40s in Germany and the experiments with Josef Mengele', the demonstrators cheered.

'That same day at a school committee meeting in North Smithfield, Rhode Island, a parent speaking against mask mandates in schools said, 'The Jews willingly got on the bus.' Despite a packed room of elected officials, educators and parents, no one called her out. At one stage, vaccine and mask refusers waved a swastika drawn from syringes outside the Massachusetts State House at an anti-vax rally featuring Republican gubernatorial candidate Geoff Diehl.

Politicians will often be quick to criticise conspiracy theorists – but perhaps sometimes there's not much difference between some of them and the people they condemn.

CHAPTER 18:

OCTOPUS VACCINES AND BABIES WITH BLACK EYES
– September 2021

▼

'CREATURE WITH TENTACLES' was the heading of the section beginning on page sixteen of the fifty-two-page report being sent by email around a group of New Hampshire politicians in the United States. The 'study' went on to detail the findings of a Dr Carrie Madej, who studied vaccine vials from Moderna and Johnson & Johnson under a high-powered 400x magnification microscope. What she saw, apparently, shocked her...

'In BOTH vials,' the report read, 'there was a living organism with tentacles. This creature moves around, lifts itself up, and even seems to be self-aware. The sight of this and the thought that these unknown, octopus-like creatures are being injected into millions of children worldwide, caused Dr Madej to weep.'

There are no living organisms in COVID-19 vaccines, but that didn't stop the theory from spinning off into the internet.

The clue to the nuttiness of the report is in its title –

'The Vaccine Death Report' – and it goes on to chronicle a list of conspiracy faves from vaccines altering the body's electromagnetic field and DNA to create a 'transhuman' without any human rights (and the slave of the person holding the patent) to the perils of 5G to the secret plan by the super-rich to rule the world. But there are some theories that stand out. One is a riff on the idea that vaccines create transhumans or, in this case, transhuman babies.

According to the report, scientists were investigating a phenomenon in Mexico where new born babies from vaccinated parents had 'pitch-black eyes' – even the whites in their eyes were black! It continues: 'It also appears that these babies are aging too fast, as they can stand and even walk at only three months old. Normally that only happens around the age of one year. Are these babies examples of transhumanism, born from parents whose DNA has been altered by gene therapy? The researchers are careful not to make premature statements but will investigate this further,' it says.

The text is accompanied by a photo of a baby, apparently sitting straight up, with unusually dark eyes. A TikTok video of the same baby went viral in 2021 and a Facebook post with the clip (now removed) read: 'Babies are being born with all black eyes, they belong to Mothers who got the jab. Don't let the government mutate your genes and your DNA.'

However, the original video from the child's proud mother, posted on 23 July 2021, showed her baby in the neonatal intensive care unit with the caption, 'less than 2 Kg can hold her head up and look at me'. The post also includes the hashtags '#pandemicbaby2020' and '#toughbaby'.

Contacted by Reuters, the baby's mother said the photo was taken several months before vaccinations began in the US, where she lives. She added that she didn't get the jab until some months after the child was born. 'I didn't take the vaccine while I was pregnant because it wasn't available for me at that time, but I did take it a few months [later],' she wrote in a Facebook message, adding: 'My baby is a very healthy baby.'

The idea that COVID vaccines can modify the DNA often stems from a controversial December 2020 paper from scientists from the prestigious Massachusetts Institute of Technology (MIT). The paper was a preprint, which means it wasn't peer-reviewed, and came under heavy fire from the scientific community even though the later, completed study never actually claimed that vaccines changed human DNA. What the researchers suggested was that the reason some people tested positive after recovering from COVID-19 was because SARS-CoV-2 could integrate pieces of its genetic code into the human genome.

Anti-vaxxers leaped on the findings to claim they related to COVID vaccines despite the authors' insistence their research had no implications for vaccines. The concern, that was soon proved justified, was that opponents of the vaccine would use the study for their own ends and use its findings out of context.

'If there ever was a preprint that should be deleted, it is this one!' said Marie-Louise Hammarskjöld, MD, PhD, a professor of microbiology at the University of Virginia, according to MedPage Today. 'It was irresponsible to even put it up as a preprint, considering the complete lack of relevant evidence. This is now being used by some to spread doubts about the new vaccines,' she added.

This seems a good time to explore exactly what is in the vaccines. There does not appear to be any strange tentacled creatures, but there is some stuff that may surprise you. The more enterprising may have checked out the side of the box before getting jabbed, but I'm guessing that the great majority did not.

For the record, there is no formaldehyde, aluminium or thimerosal (a mercury-containing organic compound sometimes used in vaccines) in either the Oxford-AstraZeneca vaccine or the Pfizer vaccine.

According to the UK government's 'Information for UK recipients on COVID-19 Vaccine' AstraZeneca, one dose (0.5 ml) of the Oxford-AstraZeneca vaccine contains the following:

COVID-19 Vaccine (ChAdOx1-S* recombinant) 5×10^{10} viral particles.

*Recombinant, replication-deficient chimpanzee adenovirus vector encoding the SARS-CoV-2 Spike glycoprotein. Produced in genetically modified human embryonic kidney (HEK) 293 cells.

This product contains genetically modified organisms (GMOs).

The other excipients are:

L-histidine

L-histidine hydrochloride monohydrate

magnesium chloride hexahydrate

polysorbate 80 (E 433)

ethanol

sucrose

sodium chloride

disodium edetate dihydrate

water for injections

Okay, so I'm no doctor but the University of Oxford Vaccine Knowledge Project offers an insight on what some of this means

(Oxford developed the vaccine with AstraZeneca). It's not actually a new technology – it's been around for about a decade – but it works by delivering SARS-CoV-2 spike protein's genetic code into the body's cells. The immune system recognises the spike protein and fights against it so that if it encounters the coronavirus spike protein in the future it will jump on it and destroy it before it can cause an infection.

The 'carrier' for the spike protein is a modified adenovirus that causes the common cold in chimpanzees, which is kind of spooky but apparently safe because it's been modified so it can't cause infection. To produce this adenovirus in the lab, according to Oxford's Vaccine Knowledge Project, the virologists used a so-called HEK-293 cell line that was taken from the kidney of a (legally) aborted foetus in 1973, although the cells used now are clones of the originals.

Now that fact is going to attract conspiracy theories, but it also represents a serious dilemma for many Catholics, who sought direction from their church.

On behalf of the bishops, the Department for Social Justice of the Catholic Bishops' Conference of England and Wales released a statement on 3 December 2020 giving its blessing to the vaccine over the thorny issue of the aborted foetus, saying: 'The Congregation for the Doctrine of the Faith and the Pontifical Academy of Life have expressed the view that one may in good conscience and for a grave reason receive a vaccine sourced in this way, provided that there is a sufficient moral distance between the present administration of the vaccine and the original wrongful action.

'In the COVID-19 pandemic, we judge that this grave reason exists and that one does not sin by receiving the vaccine ... Each Catholic must educate his or her conscience on this matter and decide what to do, also bearing in mind that a vaccine must be safe, effective and universally available, especially to the poor of the world.'

The Oxford vaccine also contains a common food additive called polysorbate 80 as an emulsifier, a small amount of alcohol (0.002 g per dose) and traces of magnesium (three to twenty parts per million).

As for the Pfizer vaccine, the UK government advice says:

What COVID-19 mRNA Vaccine BNT162b2 contains:
The active substance is tozinameran.
After dilution, the vial contains six doses, of 0.3 mL with 30 micrograms tozinameran each.
This vaccine contains polyethylene glycol/macrogol (PEG) as part of ALC-0159

The other ingredients are:
ALC-0315 = (4-hydroxybutyl)azanediyl)bis(hexane-6,1-diyl)bis(2-hexyldecanoate)
ALC-0159 = 2[(polyethylene glycol)-2000]-N,N-ditetradecylacetamide
1,2-Distearoyl-sn-glycero-3-phosphocholine
cholesterol
potassium chloride
potassium dihydrogen phosphate
sodium chloride
disodium hydrogen phosphate dihydrate
sucrose
water for injections

No chimps involved here, but the vaccine uses the genetic code (mRNA) of the spike protein from the surface of the SARS-CoV-2 virus to do the same job, faking the immune system into action so it's fired up and ready to act if it comes across it again. The active ingredient, or carrier, containing the genetic code and teaching the body how to combat COVID is the synthetically engineered 'messenger' BNT162b2, which is inside a protective fat capsule (which is where the cholesterol comes in).

The sucrose (sugar) protects the vaccine as a stabiliser when it is frozen in storage and the salts (sodium chloride, potassium chloride, potassium dihydrogen phosphate, disodium hydrogen phosphate dihydrate) help balance out the acid and alkaline balance before injection.

Rather than the old-fashioned approach of injecting a minuscule dose of the actual antigen into the body to provoke a response from the immune system, both these new COVID vaccines deliver the genetic instructions telling the body to make the antigen to cause the immune system's fightback. It is this part of the process that has been seized on by some conspiracy theorists to claim that the body's DNA is being modified by the vaccines for nefarious purposes.

The Oxford Vaccine Information Project insists that is impossible. With the mRNA (messenger Ribonucleic Acid) Pfizer vaccine, it argues that our DNA (Deoxy Ribonucleic Acid) cannot leave the nucleus of a cell and while the mRNA created to make the spike protein is delivered into the cell in a fat membrane or capsule it cannot get to the nucleus or fuse with the DNA. In other words, the human DNA is translated in a one-way process to human mRNA which is translated into human proteins.

With the Oxford vaccine, says the project, the genetic information inside the chimp adenovirus is a piece of double-stranded DNA containing the spike protein gene that urges the manufacture of the protein that stimulates the immune system into action. But with the case of the COVID vaccine, the viral gene required to replicate viral DNA has been removed, so it cannot make more viruses or cause disease. 'Such design features alongside a cell's natural DNA protection measures, prevents any possibility of viral DNA integrating with human DNA,' it adds.

Either way, the process doesn't change the body's cells. Advocates also argue that both vaccines have been successfully tested on tens of thousands of people.

Science lesson over. Back to 'The Vaccine Death Report' and its smörgåsbord of conspiracy theories about COVID, which included a claim that the millions who died in the 1918 Spanish flu outbreak were only those who had been vaccinated. It also claims that 'criminal families' operate from untouchable 'states within nations' to create a Satanist 'New World Order' – these states supposedly include Vatican City, as well as "The City of London' (an independent state within London that evades all British laws but controls the British government), and 'Washington D.C.' (or the District of Columbia, which is a sovereign state inside the United States, that rules over the American people).'

This secret cabal includes the usual names, Bill Gates (what did he do to deserve all this?), the Rothschilds, the Clintons, the Bushes, George Soros, Klaus Schwab and a couple of new ones – the shadowy 'Luciferians' in the Catholic Church, the 'Black Pope' and the 'Grey Pope'.

'It's all one huge puppet theatre, where the majority of the people – even most of those who are complicit – haven't got the slightest clue what is going on, and how everyone is being played,' the report says.

You really couldn't make this up. Actually, yes, I suppose you can...

The Republican New Hampshire state senator who circulated this report resigned from two committees after it emerged that he had disseminated the document to colleagues. He said he hadn't read it all, but acknowledged it contained 'conspiracy material'.

Back in London, the lockdown was proving just how gullible people could be. Amused by the amount of misinformation spread during the pandemic, Billy McLean, a software salesman, sent a jokey post to his mates about a novel way to feed Londoners who were self-isolating.

'My sister, her boyfriend's brother works for the Ministry of Defence and one of the things that they're doing to prepare ... is building a massive lasagne. At the moment, as we speak, they're building the massive lasagne sheets.

'They're putting the underground heating at Wembley on, that's going to bake the lasagne, and then they're putting the roof across and that's going to recreate the oven, and then what they're going to do is lift it up with drones and cut off little portions and drop it off to people's houses.'

McLean sent the WhatsApp message about the world's biggest lasagne to about thirty friends he plays football with – and it boomeranged back to him in his inbox by the end of the day after going viral across the country. 'It was just a one take,' he told the *Guardian*. 'I sent it to the football group, my mum and the girl that I'm trying to date. It went around the football group. Then I got people that I know forwarding it to me, not knowing it was me, or forwarding it to me asking if I'd heard it. Ex-girlfriends were coming out of the woodwork asking was it me.'

Some of the conspiracy theories coming out of COVID could

be pretty complex and require an expert to get into the weeds and work out their worth. You wouldn't think the great lasagne conspiracy would need a fact check. But interest in the message became so widespread that the media caught wind of it and the Football Association was forced to issue an official denial. No, it did not have any intention of turning England's soccer showplace into a giant lasagne bowl.

McLean said the prank highlighted the dangers of spreading unsubstantiated information during the pandemic. 'The intentions are good, but the outcome most of the time is pretty bad; it makes people panic more. There's no validation for what's being said in the messages. If someone sitting at home in their boxers selling software can save a one-minute clip and make it go viral, you've got to be aware that anyone can put anything out and it might not be valid.'

He may not have realised it, but the twenty-nine-year-old salesman had started something. It wasn't long before social media was abuzz with reports that the French were building a giant garlic bread in the Channel Tunnel and the Italians were tossing an enormous salad in the Coliseum in Rome!

Some other viral rumours had more serious consequences and, like the lasagne WhatsApp message, once they were out there, they were hard to rein back in.

In early March as the harsh reality of life in the pandemic was beginning to become apparent, a set of grainy photos of tanks and military vehicles in the streets started doing the rounds on social media with messages like this one, grabbed from Facebook by the BBC: 'My friend said about the army thing, I just spoke to a customer at work and he has a friend in parliament that's his source. They've got the army out already and preparing for a lockdown Friday. For fifteen days. They won't announce it until

Thurs night cos they don't want people to panic. He said they're going to be seriously strict about everything. Supermarkets are going to be open only certain hours of the day and there will be police outside it. There's gonna be police everywhere. You're gonna have to prove where you are and how urgent it is.'

Time would tell, of course, that the tanks weren't out in the streets, although the military did later deploy to help the NHS with logistics. A closer look at some of the photos also showed that the convoys were on the wrong side of the road (i.e. from Europe/America) or from before the pandemic.

Similarly, a message claiming bodies were piled up in ice rinks terrified the British public, especially as it had the veneer of authenticity because the voice of a woman claiming to work for the South East Coast Ambulance Service said hundreds of healthy children would die each day. Although one ice rink in Widnes, Cheshire, was briefly used to store bodies and there were contingency plans for temporary mortuaries, there was no truth to the claims. Nevertheless, the public response was such that Public Health England released a statement calling it 'fake news'.

Vladimir Putin may be capable of many things but releasing hundreds of lions to force Russians to stay inside and keep to lockdown rules seemed a little extreme, even for him. But a bogus tweet showing a doctored photo of a lion prowling the empty streets with the caption, 'Vladmir [sic] Putin has dropped 800 Tigers and lions all over the country to push people to stay home' was believed by many around the world. Comments on social media included posts like, 'Soooo what happens when the quarantine is over' and, 'What the??? Oh my god.'

Lord Sugar tweeted the 'Breaking News' story with the photo of the lion with the question, 'Is this a wind up?' Another

Twitter user wrote: 'Russian President Vladimir Putin has given Russians two options. You stay at home for 2 weeks or you go to jail for 5 years. The President has released 500 lions and tigers on the streets of Russia to push people to stay Home. We need a president like this Man.'

A reverse image search on Google quickly showed the photo dated back to 2016 when a lion called Columbus was snapped roaming around a Johannesburg car park.

Pranksters used the same do-it-yourself breaking news site to promote the ridiculous idea that cocaine prevented people from getting COVID. 'Live,' boasted the post, which claimed the 'Breaking News' was that 'Cocaine Kills Coronavirus – Scientist is shocked to discover that this drug can fight the virus'. A tweet with the image attached was shared thousands of times.

Another post showed a set of test results:

Cocaine – POSITIVE

Opiates – POSITIVE

Benzodiazepines – POSITIVE

Cannabis-10 – POSITIVE

COVID-19 – NEGATIVE

The 'cocaine cure' theory gained such traction in France that in March 2020, the French Government tweeted: 'No, cocaine does NOT protect against COVID-19. It is an addictive drug that causes serious side effects and is harmful to people's health.'

An unlikely winner from the pandemic were sex toy manufacturers who have seen 30 per cent to 100 per cent increases in sales and while there was little truth in rumours that masturbation was a way to prevent COVID, most experts agreed it couldn't hurt, either. In fact, New York Health Department issued guidelines during the city's first stay-at-home order that read: 'You are your safest sex partner. Masturbation will not spread COVID-19, especially if you wash your hands (and any sex toys) with soap and water for at least twenty seconds before and after sex.'

There was a less enthusiastic response to claims in India that cow dung and urine helped cure COVID-19. A popular Twitter post shows a Dr Manoj Mittal from Haryana, India, picking up a piece of dung from the ground in a field of cows and chewing on it while extolling its virtues. He clearly wasn't alone because in May 2021, Sohel Daria and Md. Rabiul Islam, from the University of Asia Pacific in Dhaka, Bangladesh, wrote an open letter published in the *International Journal of Health Planning and Management* titled, 'The use of cow dung and urine to cure COVID-19 in India: A public health concern'.

They wrote that the Hindu majority in India uses 'cow dung and urine for their wellness and cure of illness since ancient times. Also, people use cow urine as medicine in India, Nepal, Myanmar and Nigeria. But this behaviour has tremendously increased in India after the entrance of the COVID-19 pandemic. Many people are consuming cow dung and urine under branded 'cow dung therapy' for COVID cure.

'In last year, dozens of Hindu activists hosted a cow urine-drinking party in India. Some members of the Hindu nationalist party demanded that cow urine and dung can prevent and cure COVID-19. Therefore, the Indian superstitious, fanatic politicians and some other leaders disseminating the propagation that cow dung can cure COVID-19 among the general religious population.

'Superstitions about the by-products of cow has got even worse in the COVID-19 pandemic situation. Many believers in India are convinced to rub their whole body with cow dung and urine, and the packs are washed off with cow milk or buttermilk when it is dried to protect them from COVID-19. They go to cow shelters once a week for this ritual with the hope that it will boost their energy levels and immunity against COVID-19. They also drink the urine of cows to boost up their immunity to fight COVID-19. Even some healthcare professionals in India participated in rituals of using cow dung and urine to ward off COVID-19.'

The authors warned of the dangers of the practice. 'There is no concrete scientific background behind the use of cow dung or urine to boost immunity against COVID-19,' they wrote. 'But significant health risks are associated with smearing or consuming these products. Other diseases can spread from the animal to humans through this process. The human body can get ring-worm, Q-fever, chlamydiosis, leptospirosis, campylobacteriosis, salmonellosis, listeriosis, yersiniosis, cryptosporidiosis, and some other infectious diseases from cattle...

'Moreover, America's top health body Centres for Disease Control (CDC) and Prevention mentioned that mucormycetes are present in animal dung. Therefore, the experts suspect a relationship between the surge in mucormycosis (black fungal disease) and the use of cow dung during the ongoing second wave of the pandemic in India. So the use of cow dung and urine might accelerate the transmission of coronavirus along with other diseases. However, cow dung and urine were the fastest-growing alternative medicine business in India.'

A more first world problem is the man claiming on TikTok that getting the Oxford-AstraZeneca shot has made him Bluetooth connectable everywhere he goes. He features in two videos that went viral before being taken off TikTok, but they remained on Instagram and Facebook, albeit with a 'false information' warning.

Sitting at the counter in the first video, the man complains that wherever he goes his body hooks up with the Bluetooth.

'I was a little sore,' he says, talking about how he felt after getting the vaccine. 'The only problem is that everywhere I go – everywhere I go – everything is starting to connect to me, man, like Bluetooth connective. I get in the car and my car is trying to connect me, I get home and my computer is trying to connect, my phone is trying to connect. I keep getting this bloody notification, look, check this out,' he says and shows the camera his phone with the screen offering to pair with a device called 'AstraZeneca_ChAdOx1-S.'

In the second, linked video, the same man says, 'The connectivity is still there, man, I don't know how to turn it off.' He can be seen walking up to a wall-mounted TV and holding up his hand until a message comes up on the screen that says: 'Connecting to AstraZeneca_ChAdOx1-S...'

'There it is,' he adds. 'Everywhere I get the same message.'

There's no evidence to suggest the AstraZeneca vaccine contains anything that might connect through Bluetooth and it's actually pretty easy to call a connectable Bluetooth device anything you want – including 'AstraZeneca_ChAdOx1-S.'

The crazier the theories, the easier it tends to be to debunk them. It's not so easy to tell who is larking around ... and who is deadly serious.

CHAPTER 19:

PANDEMIC, WHAT PANDEMIC?
– September 2021

▼

It was the kind of beautiful summer's evening your grandparents told you doesn't happen any more. A slight breeze in the sloping meadow shimmering through the grass all the way down to the sea mirroring the darkening sky above. In the United Kingdom, you learn to treasure these long nights as the softening light turns down the heat to dusk and you file the sunshine away in your memory to talk about one day with the grandkids.

Parked at the top of a field facing the ocean in Padstow, Cornwall, in September 2021, it was easy to forget there had been a pandemic. When you are travelling in a bright orange 1972 VW camper van called Blossom there is no need for social distancing and no room for paranoia.

The open road was a welcome relief from the constraints of COVID and there were just four other families in the remote field, a small price to pay for a longer walk to the bathroom. One of them, two spaces back but with no less of a view, was camped around a blue VW camper of similar vintage. Like motorcycle riders, VW owners share a wave or a smile on the road and so it seemed only natural for our campsite neighbour to pay us a friendly visit.

He was an older man dressed in tweed and a checked shirt that looked like it came straight from the shelves at Gieves & Hawkes, maybe a grandfather himself judging by the ages of the children playing by his van, and we shared a pleasant few minutes discussing the dexterity/contortions required in steering these old machines through the narrow Cornish lanes.

And then, inevitably, the conversation turned to COVID.

I'd become used to avoiding controversial topics such as whether people are vaccinated or agreed with wearing masks – they usually told you anyway pretty much straight away – but I felt on safe ground with this old gentleman. If a marketing company were to draw up a portrait of a patriotic, double-vaxxed and boosted, stickler for the rules then he was your man. Maybe he had a few qualms about the government's handling of the whole thing but that was okay. Who doesn't? Besides, he mentioned when we met that he worked 'somewhere in Whitehall'. I don't know why but it felt reassuring when he said it. Like he knew stuff we didn't and look at him out here in the sunshine with his family as if nothing had happened.

But then, and this took a while to seep into my sun-addled mind, it became apparent that he actually didn't believe anything had happened. The pandemic was 'an excuse', he said, without explaining why. He started peppering my wife and me with questions...

'Do you know anyone who has died of COVID?'

'Well, no, but er...'

'Did you know that the hospitals were all empty?'

'Well, no, but er...'

'Did you know they only want to vaccinate us to keep tabs on what we're doing?'

'Well, no, but er...'

He was a walking, talking conspiracy theorist from Dorking, Surrey. The stockbroker belt. About as far from a trendy, green hippie as you could possibly get. This old man wasn't sitting in his underpants on the Internet into the early hours of the morning, eating cold pizza and sharing dark visions of a cyber-conspiracy. He wasn't drinking the Kool-Aid on Hampstead Heath with a bunch of New Age travellers. He was in the garden cutting back rose bushes and chatting over the fence with his next-door neighbour. Before popping back inside for a cup of tea and a ginger biscuit, they'd chat about how the COVID-19 pandemic was a lot of old poppycock.

It was a sobering lesson. If there once was a trust in government, it has been eroded over time to such an extent that ordinary people – decent, family people – were questioning what they were told, and some had clearly come to the conclusion they were being lied to, to the extent that some believed COVID never really happened.

Mention the words conspiracy theories in the UK and the first name that is likely to spring to mind is David Icke, the former footballer and BBC sports broadcaster turned bizarro theorist-in-chief who believes the world is secretly run by shape-shifting reptiles from outer space and that the Royal Family are lizards. It was no surprise to anybody when Icke jumped on the COVID bandwagon, essentially telling his 382,000 Twitter followers (until he was barred from using the platform in November 2020) and 900,000 YouTube subscribers (until his channel was deleted in May 2020) that the pandemic was 'a load of nonsense'.

Icke sees COVID, and indeed, Russia's invasion of Ukraine, as steps to dismantle Western civilisation and global warming as a 'ludicrous hoax'. Before COVID, he saw the West as paying 'lip service' to democracy while China, which he sees as a guinea pig for the rest of the world, experimented with autocratic control in real time. With a 'woke' President Biden in place in the US, he saw COVID as a way the psychopathic elite could reframe the world in China's image as a 'Hunger Games' society with a tiny few at the top controlling the subservient masses. By manipulating the public with 'fake' vaccines and mandates, these 'psychopaths' as he calls them, have tricked people into giving up their rights to free thought and created a new mindset of subservience.

To Icke and his ilk, the pandemic was manna from heaven, feeding directly into their new world order conspiracy theories. Icke's views are probably a little too wacky for my campsite neighbour in Cornwall, but, honestly, I'm not absolutely sure of that. An interviewer on one podcast said he used to smoke large quantities of marijuana and sit around with his mates watching David Icke videos for 'entertainment' and that sounds about right to me. Icke was laughed off after first airing some of his views on Terry Wogan's prime time BBC chat show in 1991 (he said the world was going to end in 1997 and claimed to be the 'son of the Godhead'). But he was identified by the Center for Countering Digital Hate as one of the world's leading spreaders of disinformation about COVID-19. The CCDH says Icke's website is one of the 1,000 most popular in the UK and claims his COVID conspiracy theories have been viewed over thirty million times on social media.

In an ultimately successful campaign to get Icke deplatformed from social media, CCDH CEO Imran Ahmed wrote: 'Taken together, his videos outline a "superconspiracy" in which COVID-19 does not exist and has been invented by a "global cult" to justify the imposition of an "Orwellian global state". Millions have watched Icke explain how Bill Gates and the Jewish Rothschilds form part of that cult, and how 5G networks and vaccines are the real cause of COVID-19. This is having real world consequences. In the UK, there was a wave of arson attacks on 5G phone masts after videos of Icke falsely linking them to COVID-19 were shared in Facebook groups, amassing millions of views. In North America, anti-lockdown protestors have cited David Icke as their inspiration.'

One video claiming the Rothschilds family was involved in planning the pandemic was viewed more than 5.9 million times, making it the twenty-seventh most popular video about coronavirus on YouTube. London Real, with 2.6 million followers, introduces Icke as 'a full-time investigator into who and what is really controlling the world'.

Icke is no joke. He may be a former goalkeeper and sports commentator with a big smile, but he has millions of followers who take his theories very seriously.

Icke's US equivalent is a more belligerent character whose conspiracy theories have a darker side.

Right-wing radio host Alex Jones claims COVID is both a hoax and a scam, although he admits to being sick with the virus early in 2022. His Infowars website has repeatedly posted misinformation about the pandemic, including claims that the vaccines were a form of gene therapy that modified a person's DNA.

His insistence that the 2012 Sandy Hook school shooting in which twenty children and six adults were killed was faked using actors to help create a case for gun control in the US led to him being sued for defamation by families of the victims. He later acknowledged in a deposition that the shootings were real.

Piers Morgan took a lot of stick in 2013 when he interviewed Jones on his CNN show and the ultraconservative radio talk show host shouted down Morgan's attempts to take him to task over gun control. Even colleague Wolf Blitzer asked the Briton: 'Were you comfortable giving [Alex Jones] all this airtime, this publicity on your show?' Apple, Facebook, Spotify and YouTube had already dropped him before the pandemic because of his 'hate speech'.

But, like Icke, Jones doesn't appear to need the mainstream media to find his followers. His YouTube channel had 2.4 million subscribers before it was canned and, according to the Huffington Post, the store on his Infowars website raked in over $165 million in three years from 2015 selling supplements and survivalist equipment.

These guys are the extremists. Icke believes in reptilian rulers and Jones insisted that many of the children killed in the Sandy Hook school massacre were actors. But what about the COVID naysayers who take a less sensationalistic approach? Should they be allowed a voice? Should we believe everything we are told?

CHAPTER 20:

CHAMPAGNE FOR BREAKFAST AND GOING AGAINST THE GRAIN

– March 2017

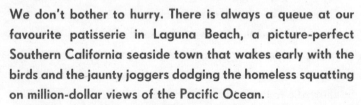

We don't bother to hurry. There is always a queue at our favourite patisserie in Laguna Beach, a picture-perfect Southern California seaside town that wakes early with the birds and the jaunty joggers dodging the homeless squatting on million-dollar views of the Pacific Ocean.

The double door at Moulins eases open and we are met first with the smell of croissants fresh out of the oven, warm chocolate just released into the pastry, almond burnt not to a crisp but just crisp, and the soft, buttery defeat of an Ottoman crescent.

They sit by the cash till, begging to be bought, but first you must battle through the wild meadow of cakes and salads behind glass cases demanding attention as you wait to be served in the long, slow line. It is the only place in California I know where patience is rewarded.

We head not to the food, still untouched by the gannets who

will pick and ravage through the day, but for the fridge packed with orange juice, energy drinks, sodas and $3 waters that will soon be snapped up by hungry runners to wash down their excuses. I reach for a half bottle of Laurent-Perrier champagne.

My wife, Michelle, leaves me to take care of the order while she snags a table on the patio. After a morning on the beach, we often roll in here in sandy swimsuits, damp sweats and tangled hair. The crêpes are a favourite with the kids and the servers are happy to step over our Siberian Husky playing dead in the entrance. But today, my wife is dressed to impress; a silky red dress falls easily off her shoulders, gathering slightly at the waist before landing just above her white espadrilles, the ties sidling out of sight along her tanned calves. Her hair is straightened and long and the slight blush on her cheeks matches her lips and sets off the knife lines of her cheekbones. She wouldn't have been out of place at Guy Savoy in Paris. I wash up well, too, in jeans and a crisp, white shirt, if only to complement my beautiful wife.

There is no judgement from the young French waitress from Paris, who is spending the summer improving her English. She simply asks if I would like an ice bucket and says she will bring the champagne to our table. I am grateful she doesn't offer to send over a cupcake with a candle or round up the servers to sing 'Joyeux Anniversaire'.

I order a quiche Lorraine and a croque monsieur with a side of French fries and because I am thinking about how much I don't want the awkwardness of a celebratory cupcake; I add a molten dark chocolate hazelnut tart for dessert. The waitress asks for my table number and is already serving the next customer as I count my change.

It is a gorgeous morning, as they invariably are in Orange County. I always joke about how much people talk about the weather in England, forgetting how rich and varied (and wet) it is. In California, you don't hear folks forecasting the week ahead; it's usually a done deal. They prefer to say they've been blessed, as if the unrelenting sunshine is their divine right.

With the tourists gone and the autumnal sun taking a more benevolent hue, the September street outside Moulins is still quiet with a handful of scraggy, blond surfers, their futures wrapped up in the tides, ambling past with boards under their arms to check on the waves breaking next to Pacific Coast Highway a short walk away.

Professional types in Teslas and Oakleys, bobs and side partings, park outside to eat on the run. The regulars remember to put money in the meters, knowing they will have to wait. The others must factor the cost of a parking ticket into their $4 croissants. We watch them knowingly, nodding occasionally to other locals.

The champagne arrives first, as it should. It opens with a loud pop and our neighbours smile, silently questioning why we would be drinking at 9:30am on a Thursday morning. We smile back.

We take our first sips of champagne, the bubbles flooding our dry, tight mouths with life, and a voice calls out our names from across the road: 'My English friends! Where's the party?'

Michael is the Laguna Beach Town Greeter. It's an honorary job he has given himself, but the tradition dates back more than 125 years and the town's most famous greeter Eiler Larsen, a shaggy-haired Danish immigrant who welcomed visitors from the 1940s to the early 1970s, has two statues in his memory. Every morning at 7am, Michael arrives at the corner of Broadway and PCH to dance and wave a greeting to passing motorists. Every afternoon, he dances outside the Sapphire restaurant up the hill at the other end of Laguna. His props are an empty plastic bottle, crushed flat so he can step on it and spin, and a small assortment of extravagant hats and outfits.

Today, he is wearing an old favourite, a red military uniform with yellow tassels and a white sailor's cap with matching gloves. In another life, he would crash Hollywood parties and be photographed with the likes of Tom Hanks, Elton John and Michael Jackson. In another life before that, he was married in Massachusetts. Now he is homeless and sleeps on the beach. He says he enjoys making other people happy, but he takes the unpaid job very seriously. He knows every local and remembers every name. He survives, not by panhandling, which he deems below the status of a town greeter, but through handouts from restaurant and shop owners. It's a small price to pay for the smiles.

Dig a little deeper and it isn't so easy. An old iPod full of music I gave him was stolen the first night from his sleeping spot on the beach and it can get bitterly cold at night, even here in paradise. He dances across the street, carrying a plastic bag containing all his belongings. 'Congratulations! Every day is champagne day in Laguna Beach.' He doesn't ask what we are celebrating. 'I just saw your daughter in Laguna Coffee. Such a lovely girl, takes after her mother.'

He takes an impossibly smooth pebble from his jacket pocket and gives it to my wife 'for luck'. She smiles, touched to tears, but I can see she doesn't want to chat.

'What are you listening to?' I ask. Michael always has his earphones in.

'Some Stones,' he says, adopting a gunslinger pose. 'I'm working on my Jagger moves.'

He waves across the restaurant. 'How ya doin', Debbie? Have a terrific day.'

'Gotta get back to work,' he says, turning back to us and then strutting away like a catwalk model. 'Moves like Jagger,' he sings over his shoulder.

The food is coming, and I notice my wife's glass is empty. I take advantage of a rare lull, running to the cashier with a second half bottle. By the time I'm back, the table is full with breakfast, fries and chocolate and I commandeer a spare chair for the champagne bucket refreshed with new ice and more bubbles. I raise a toast and we share a look. 'To the future,' I say.

We both go to say something, but the look seems to have said it all. We dig into our breakfasts listening to the door opening and closing behind us.

The croque and the quiche really are delicious, but we don't manage the chocolate hazelnut tart. We decide to leave after the owner, arriving from one of his other patisseries, sees us and the two upturned champagne bottles.

'I love you guys,' he says. 'You know how to live like the French. If you want champagne in the morning, you drink it. Why wait until lunchtime? This must be the third time this week.'

He pats my shoulder, kisses Michelle on the cheek and goes inside. She carefully wraps the uneaten tart in a napkin, gathers up her coat and waits for me to finish my champagne.

It is, indeed, the third time this week. The third champagne breakfast, the third visit to hospital and the third time we have stopped the whirlwind long enough to breathe.

In the first hospital visit, the cancer nurses trialled a new biopsy needle on my wife and kept jabbing at the lump in her breast until she cried out for them to please stop. I wasn't allowed in with her and my heart broke the moment she walked into the waiting room, her pale, elfin face filled with pain.

We went to Moulins that morning and ordered champagne. Then we called the children to tell them the worst.

The second visit we saw the surgeon together. He was young and all-American, and his name was Washington. The tumour was the size of a lacrosse ball (slightly smaller than a tennis ball), he said, and he had scheduled an operation to remove it the following week. There would be chemo and radiation and drugs, and it was all arranged. He was certain. He didn't entertain any doubts.

We went straight to Moulins and ordered champagne. That was a full bottle.

The third hospital visit was just as devastating. The cosmetic surgeon was a woman and she, too, was certain. It would have to be a mastectomy. The tumour was simply too large for anything else, and it would be at least a year before she could start any reconstruction. She dropped these bombs in between checking her phone and her tweets and taking calls. She had the bedside manner of Harold Shipman.

And so here we are again, drinking champagne as our world collapses around us. We raise a glass to the French poet, Paul Claudel, who wrote: 'In the little moment that remains to us between the crisis and the catastrophe, we may as well drink a glass of champagne.' And my movie buff wife quotes Bette Davis who, as Kit Marlowe in *Old Acquaintance*, said: 'There comes a time in every woman's life when the only thing that helps is a glass of champagne.' We'd laughed over these sayings before but neither of us is laughing now.

This moment is all we can be sure of, the first sip of champagne, and with it the memories of all the celebrations from times past. The courting, the passion, the contentment, the wedding, the births, the birthdays, the Christmases, the bright summer evenings overlooking a darkening ocean with a fleet of pelicans in a V-shaped shadow across the red sky and a glass of champagne to celebrate absolutely nothing other than life together, uncomplicated and for ever.

We have little faith in the doctors and their cutting and their poison and their certainties. We don't believe in their prognosis or in the future they are planning for us that can so easily be erased. But we do have now, the next minute, and the next. We will not keep our champagne on ice.

My wife sits back down and gets the chocolate hazelnut tart out of her bag, carefully unwrapping it back on to the plate. There's that look again, the one that says in an instant everything that has passed between us in a quarter-century of marriage.

And I head inside to buy another bottle of Laurent-Perrier, knowing for certain that tomorrow can wait a little longer...

This happened to us five years ago in the days after my wife's first cancer prognosis. We still drink the occasional glass of champagne, although rarely with breakfast (at least, not without a splash of orange juice) to celebrate the tomorrows that continue to come despite the warnings of her doctors.

I include it for a reason, to explain how ordinary people – people like us – no longer believe the opinion of the medical profession is sacrosanct. Anyone with kids will wonder why the same antibiotic is doled out for a kaleidoscope of differing ailments; anyone in their sixties and beyond may well wonder why their health issues largely revolve around the harm done to their bodies by years of steroids, antibiotics and other chemicals prescribed to 'heal' long-forgotten illnesses and conditions.

And anyone who has had cancer may wonder why their bodies were poisoned and burned in the name of a 'cure'.

Nevertheless, many who choose conventional chemotherapy and radiation treatments also have good reasons to be grateful to their doctors for helping them navigate through their darkest times.

My wife's decision to reject traditional medicine's methods of treating breast cancer and focusing on alternative treatments has been a long and lonely road with little support from our healthcare provider when we were living in the US, or the National Health Service in the UK. The truth is that most oncologists and medical professionals we have come into contact with in these vast organisations have no time for anyone who questions the conventional chemo-based treatments. They are blunt and matter of fact. There was only one option for treatment – theirs. There was only one outcome if my wife rejected their recommendations. She would die.

As I mentioned, that was five years ago...

Fast-forward to COVID and the medical profession has come into question as never before. The internet has allowed us a window into the make-up of the virus and the diverse ways that different countries and communities have dealt with the pandemic. We have information that was denied from previous generations that had little choice but to trust in the doctors, scientists and politicians who decided on their fate. If bad decisions were made it was unlikely they would have ever known about them, let alone raised questions.

COVID was different. The longer the pandemic continued, the more frayed the public trust became, especially when Downing Street advisor Dominic Cummings drove to his father's farm in Durham during a lockdown in May 2020 and then Prime Minister Boris Johnson attended a Christmas party at Number 10 at a time in December 2020 when the rest of the country was being implored by the government to stay at home.

No right-minded people would criticise the doctors, nurses and first responders who risked their lives and worked long hours to help those afflicted by this terrible virus and it is ridiculous to suggest the pandemic was a figment of the government and media elite's fertile imagination.

We should understand, too, that change is at the very heart of science; it is rarely exact. Scientists, especially those at the cutting edge, are often learning as they go along and adapting their methods and their sometimes-changing path. It was hardly surprising that leaders who claimed to be 'following the science' in their handling of the pandemic would make so many false steps.

But serious people were asking serious questions about how the virus was being handled and there was an avalanche of theories about how the crisis should be handled. With every government misstep, the distrust grew.

In a conversation with *The Atlantic* editor Jeffrey Goldberg on 6 April, former President Barack Obama admitted he had underestimated the 'demand for crazy' online and criticised social media's role in spreading disinformation.

'I grappled with it a lot during my presidency, and I saw it unfold,' he said of the way information and disinformation was being weaponised. 'We saw it, but I think I underestimated the degree to which democracies were as vulnerable to it as they were, including ours.'

Obama acknowledged that many Americans were tuning out the facts. 'Unfiltered, there's literally nothing you can't receive in this room right now,' he said, 'and yet, in our society, you have roughly 40 per cent of the country that appears convinced that the current president was elected fraudulently and that the election was rigged, and you have 30 to 35 per cent of the country that has chosen not to avail itself of a medical miracle, the development of a vaccine faster than anything we have ever seen before, which, by the way, has now been tested by about a billion people and yet are still refusing to take it despite extraordinary risks to themselves and their families.

'Misinformation is just wrong information and that's always been with us,' he continued. 'We get facts wrong; we say stuff wrong, and we are not going to solve that problem any time soon. The way I define disinformation is if you have a systematic effort to either promote false information, to suppress true information for the purpose of political gain, financial gain, enhancing power, suppressing others, targeting those you don't like and that I think is entirely different from information that is inconvenient.'

Obama lamented the demise of local newspapers, replaced by online outlets with fewer checks and balances and quoted a study in which 'hard core conservative' Fox News-watching participants were paid to watch CNN. 'In a relatively short period of time what it showed was that their views on controversial issues like immigration or police or vaccinations had changed by 5 or 8 or 10 per cent, just simply by changing their diet. It hadn't turned them into liberals, it didn't make them want to vote for Joe Biden. They had just had access to a different set of information. I say that to suggest that we underestimate the degree of pliability in our opinions and our views.

'It does give me faith that if people are given different information they can process differently.'

Obama described himself as being close to an 'absolutist' on free speech and believes that uncomfortable topics should be debated. But he said big tech, as private companies, are already making key decisions about what appears on their platforms and should face some regulations to discourage 'toxic' information from being spread.

Leading anti-vaxxers – not as extreme as the likes of Icke and Jones but sceptical about the reasoning and the science behind lockdowns, masks, vaccinations and the handling of the pandemic – believe the social media giants are already overplaying their censorship hands.

Former *New York Times* journalist Alex Berenson was permanently banned from Twitter after questioning the COVID vaccine in a tweet that was flagged by the social media giant. The Yale-educated writer – who had over 340,000 followers – posted a screen shot of the offending message together with a note reading: 'This was the tweet that did it. Entirely accurate. I can't wait to hear what a jury will make of this.'

The post questioned the insistence by the US Centers of Disease Control and Prevention, backed by clinical trials, that the COVID vaccines were 'safe and effective'.

'It doesn't stop infection. Or transmission,' wrote Berenson. 'Don't think of it as a vaccine,' he continued. 'Think of it – at best – as a therapeutic with a limited window of efficacy and terrible side effect profile that must be dosed IN ADVANCE OF ILLNESS.'

Now you can agree with Berenson or vehemently disagree. You can call him a conspiracy theorist, if you like (he says he is not), but the point is whether anonymous employees at social media companies should have the power to curtail free speech? And if they do, where will it end? With Elon Musk's proposed purchase of Twitter, that grey area became even greyer.

Berenson, writing in the *Wall Street Journal* on 7 December

2020, accused Amazon of suppressing self-published booklets he had written that challenged measures taken to control the pandemic.

'Information has never been more plentiful or easier to distribute,' he wrote. 'Yet we are sliding into a new age of censorship and suppression, encouraged by technology giants and traditional media companies. As someone who's been falsely characterised as a coronavirus "denier", I have seen this crisis first-hand.'

He claimed that at least half a dozen authors had their books pulled even though Amazon sold Hitler's *Mein Kampf* and *The Anarchist's Cookbook*. He also alleged YouTube had taken down over 200,000 videos about the pandemic, including one by a doctor advising then President Trump.

'Facebook has not only censored videos and attached warning labels or "fact checks" to news articles but removed groups that oppose lockdowns and other restrictions,' he wrote, adding: 'That online entertainment and retail companies have benefited financially from lockdowns adds to the ugliness of their suppression efforts.'

Berenson also accused the mainstream media of stifling debate over COVID, saying they were 'unwilling even to ask ideologically inconvenient questions'.

'Fortunately, business leaders like Elon Musk and indepen-dent-thinking media figures like Glenn Greenwald came to my defence. Amazon eventually relented. But many other people and ideas are still being suppressed,' he continued.

At the heart of the debate is who should decide what the public should know and when would an intervention be appropriate. It is interesting to note which countries ban Twitter and Facebook; the answer is China, North Korea,

Iran and Turkmenistan. In early March 2022 – soon after invading Ukraine – Russia joined that list, citing 'fake' reports about the war.

Another case in point is the lab leak theory that was so long discredited as a conspiracy theory. In May 2021, Facebook decided to lift its ban on posts suggesting the virus was man-made or manufactured 'in light of ongoing investigations into the origin'.

Just three months earlier, Facebook said any posts about a lab leak would be blocked, saying: 'Following consultations with leading health organizations, including the World Health Organization (WHO), we are expanding the list of false claims we will remove to include additional debunked claims about the coronavirus and vaccines.'

Nick Hudson, chairman of PANDA (Pandemics Data & Analytics), a group of multi-disciplinary professionals worried about the 'overwrought' response to COVID-19, and the lockdown mandates in particular, found himself permanently banned from Twitter and his 64,000 followers in March 2022 after tweeting an 'offhand remark' about the anti-parasitic drug ivermectin, a controversial early treatment for COVID.

'We have seen governments instructing big tech firms to preserve a narrative,' Hudson said in an interview on Substack. 'It's not a requirement that they demonstrate that something you say is false, they simply need to demonstrate, or just say, that it contradicts what is being said by the government.'

Hudson's opposition to the mask mandate in his native South Africa had led to an earlier twelve-hour Twitter ban. The offending tweet read: 'So South Africans, it's your duty to frustrate the mask mandate at every opportunity. The stupid things don't work. The scientists who say they do are all corrupt so ignore them. Let's erode this by following the example of our townships which have had no compliance since last year.'

'The interesting thing about this,' added Hudson, 'is that now statements about mask inefficacy have become pretty much widespread and you even hear them from mainstream scientists. In South Africa, we have scientists who have been at the forefront of rolling out the COVID malarkey acknowledging that, in the one case the guy came out and said that listen, they are there for theatre, to remind people of the presence of a deadly virus. So, do we consider them wrong, now those mainstream scientists agree with me, and it seems like everybody agrees, or there's at least been a shift towards this perspective? Nine months ago, it was contravening policy. Many people out there are unaware of the degree of censorship, both in media and in social media that is prevalent,' he told interviewer Sonia Elijah, who said: 'It's very frightening. We are supposed to be living in a democracy. We're not living in China.'

Perhaps the root of the answer may lie in a less absolutist attitude from the medical profession that has lost its godlike status with the rise of WebMD and other health information websites.

My wife is not a public figure; she's not looking to make a fuss. She just wants doctors and specialists to listen to her and respect her opinion. And maybe even help her. That doesn't seem to be too much to ask from a profession that routinely took out children's tonsils before discovering it led to twice to three times as many upper respiratory tract diseases. They don't do it much any more, especially because your tonsils produce immune cells that produce antibodies that kill viruses like COVID before they can hurt the rest of the body. They don't do lobotomies either. Medicine, like science, is an ever-changing, ever-evolving discipline. Treatments for COVID will evolve, just as they will for cancer.

Primum non nocere, or 'First, do no harm', is an important principle in medicine and, as long as the debate adheres to that oath, people with conflicting opinions and beliefs should be encouraged to ask their questions without being dismissed as troublemakers or conspiracy theorists. They don't even have to be right, just sincere and authentic and cognisant of how their arguments may influence others. By ignoring people with legitimate concerns, way more harm may be done in the long run.

As Winston Churchill said, 'Perhaps it is better to be irresponsible and right, than to be responsible and wrong.'

CHAPTER 21:

RFK & THE DISINFORMATION DOZEN
– February–March 2021

His father and his uncles are the focus of some of history's most famous conspiracy theories. Robert F. Kennedy Jr. was nine years old when his uncle, President John F. Kennedy was assassinated in 1963 and fourteen when his father, Robert F. Kennedy, was shot dead five years later.

He would have known about the unanswered questions swirling over these iconic assassinations from an early age, just as he would know about the mystery over Uncle Teddy's 1969 car crash on Chappaquiddick Island that left a young woman, Mary Jo Kopechne, dead.

Did Lee Harvey Oswald really act alone when he shot JFK in Dallas? Did Sirhan Sirhan have an accomplice in a polka-dot dress when he gunned down RFK in Los Angeles? Why did Teddy Kennedy wait so long to tell police he had been unable to save his woman passenger after driving off a bridge near Martha's Vineyard?

Now here's a new question for aficionados of America's tumultuous first family – how did a scion of the storied political dynasty come to be accused of being one of the notorious Disinformation Dozen?

According to the London-based Center for Countering Digital Hate, a non-profit that targets social media over its failures to tackle racism and anti-vaccine propaganda online, an overwhelming majority of the conspiracy theories about COVID and anti-vaccine disinformation originate from just twelve people.

Of 812,000 Facebook posts and tweets analysed by the CCDH between 1 February and 16 March 2021, 65 per cent of them came from the 'Disinformation Dozen'. On Facebook alone during that period, they accounted for 73 per cent of all anti-vaxxer content.

'This shows that while many people might spread anti-vaccine content on social media platforms, the content they share often comes from a much more limited range of sources,' said the CCDH in its report, 'The Disinformation Dozen: Why Platforms Must Act on Twelve Leading Online Anti-Vaxxers'. 'Exposure to even a small amount of online vaccine misinformation has been shown by the Vaccine Confidence Project to reduce the number of people willing to take a COVID vaccine by up to 8.8 per cent,' it adds.

The same twelve are said to be responsible for up to 17 per cent of 120,000 anti-vaxxer tweets sent during the 1 February–16 March test period.

'With the vast majority of harmful content being spread by a select number of accounts, removing those few most dangerous individuals and groups can significantly reduce the amount of disinformation being spread across platforms,' the CCDH report concludes in its demand for the twelve to be deplatformed. 'The public cannot make informed decisions about their health when they are constantly inundated by disinformation and false content. By removing the source of disinformation, social media platforms including Facebook, Instagram and Twitter can enable individuals to make a truly informed choice about vaccines,' it adds.

The report puts RFK Jr. at number 2 in its top twelve hit list, calling him 'a long-standing anti-vaxxer'. It adds that his Children's Health Defense website hosts 'a range of anti-vaccine articles' and released a film in mid-March 2021 'targeting members of the Black and Latino communities with tailored anti-vaccine messages'.

Tortoise news site also analysed 145,000 Instagram and Facebook posts with 'verified' disinformation and found that Kennedy's posts had the biggest impact. 'Kennedy Jr is one of the main anti-vax voices out there,' Tim Caulfield, professor of health law and science policy at the University of Alberta, told Tortoise. 'He comes with some credibility with his name and the work he's done in the environmental space. He's more likely to get a seat at the table and be viewed as a credible voice.'

The third of RFK and Ethel Kennedy's eleven children is an environmental law specialist and already had a fierce reputation before the pandemic as a vaccine naysayer. His opposition to vaccines by linking them to autism and other conditions such as attention deficit hyperactivity disorders and food allergies prompted his siblings Joseph P. Kennedy and Kathleen Kennedy Townsend and niece Maeve Kennedy McKean to go public with their concerns during the 2019 measles outbreak, writing in Politico that he was 'part of a misinformation campaign that's having heart-breaking – and deadly – consequences'.

Unbowed by the criticism, RFK Jr. has refused to back down over his warnings about vaccinations during the pandemic.

In a 6 August 2021 Instagram Live interview with actor Alec Baldwin and his 1.8 million Instagram followers, he said he 'stumbled' into vaccine hesitancy in 2005 after American mothers drew his attention to the mercury that was then in some vaccines. 'It's not something I want to be doing ... but I know too much,' he said.

He said he asked top experts back then how the US Centers for Disease Control could warn pregnant mothers against eating tuna fish sandwiches while also recommending a flu shot that contains mercury (as a preservative) that is going to expose a foetus to 'much higher doses than eating 50 tuna fish sandwiches a week'.

'None of them could answer that question,' he said.

'I think COVID is real and it's a horrible, baffling illness,' said Kennedy, who was promoting therapeutic treatments such as hydroxychloroquine and immune boosters over vaccinations. 'It's doing things that are really unpredictable and I don't think we really understand the mechanisms,' he told Baldwin.

Kennedy claimed authorities should do more 'risk assessment' to determine the human cost of strategies such as quarantines and lockdowns and quoted a report that claimed every additional point rise in unemployment led to more deaths, more suicides and more cases of people entering mental institutions. 'One thing I think we're not thinking about is what is the death toll from the quarantine,' he claimed, adding: 'The death toll from quarantine could far exceed the death toll from COVID.'

He also claimed that statistics were being twisted in the UK. 'In Britain, in five weeks during April and May, you had 30,000 additional deaths, excess deaths, in nursing homes,' he told Baldwin. 'There were more than 30,000 more deaths than expected. But when they went and looked, they found that only 10,000 of those people had COVID; 20,000 of them died because they weren't getting their kidney dialysis, because they were getting heart attacks and weren't getting treated. Isolation kills people too,' he added.

Kennedy said a lot of people were unhappy because of the lack of debate over the options in handling COVID. 'That debate is not happening on CNN or any of the places we go for news,' he said. 'It's all about the pharmaceutical paradigm, do what you're told, believe what we tell you and I think it polarises people and makes them angry and it makes them say, "I'm not going to do what you tell me because you're not explaining to me the truth, you're not allowing this debate to happen, you're not persuading me."'

He continued: 'In a democracy, we want leadership, but we don't want bullying. That is why I think a lot of people are resisting masks and stuff ... Americans are people who want to make sacrifices, but they don't want to be ordered what to do.'

It's worth noting that in the first few months of the pandemic, Kennedy's social media following tripled from 229,000 followers to 665,000 and he won support for his controversial views from Hollywood stars like Robert De Niro and Jim Carrey. The Kennedy cachet was having an impact.

Kennedy finished the conversation with Baldwin by telling him: 'I hope you don't take too much crap for talking to me. You've got a lot of courage.' He knew all too well that the interview was enough to cause a backlash against the actor and he was right. Baldwin took a bashing on Twitter for not confronting Kennedy over some of his controversial views while others praised him for giving the VIP anti-vaxxer a platform.

Professor Peter Hotez, a vaccine scientist at Texas' Baylor University, blasted Baldwin in a tweet for the interview, writing: 'Always disappointing when celebrities go out of their way to advertise their ignorance and promote anti-science conspiracy theories, especially during these troubled times.'

Hugely popular podcast host Joe Rogan would face an even bigger backlash more than a year later after a group of 270 doctors and health experts wrote an open letter to Spotify, the music streaming service that paid a reputed $200 million for Rogan's services, complaining about bogus medical advice they said he was giving his audience and his choice of some conspiracy theory guests.

'Mass-misinformation events of this scale have extraordinarily dangerous ramifications,' they wrote about Rogan's show, which was drawing about eleven million listeners per episode. Musicians Neil Young, Joni Mitchell, David Crosby and Stephen Stills all then boycotted the platform over Rogan's content.

The conundrum remained; how do you allow free speech while preventing possibly harmful disinformation?

The CCDH will argue that by stopping the supply, the demand will dry up. But the substantial audiences for the remaining eleven members of the Disinformation Dozen may disagree.

Top of the list at number one is Joseph Mercola, who is described by the CCDH as a 'successful anti-vaccine entrepreneur, peddling dietary supplements and false cures as alternatives to vaccines'. His combined personal social media accounts were said in the CCDH report to total around 3.6 million followers. He prefers to describe himself as helping people 'taking charge of our own health'.

While Mercola has long attracted a big audience attracted to his alternative health views and products, his extreme views on COVID treatments earned him the title in the *New York Times* as 'the most influential spreader of coronavirus misinformation online'.

One article alone calling vaccines a 'medical fraud' and alleging they 'alter your genetic coding, turning you into a viral protein factory that has no off-switch', reached over 400,000 people on Facebook, according to *The Times*.

The osteopathic physician from Cape Coral, Florida, is said to have a net worth of $100 million as a result of his natural health empire. Examples of his disinformation 'violations' in the CCDH report include a tweet that reads: 'The same number of people have died in 2020 that, on average, have died in previous years. This simply wouldn't be the case if we had a lethal pandemic.'

Another example of a so-called disinformation 'violation' turned out to be prescient. It reads: 'Forced vaccination is part of the plan to "reset" the global economic system. Now, global vaccine passports are being introduced, and it's only a matter of time before vaccination status will be a prerequisite for travel.'

After Robert F. Kennedy Jr., Ty and Charlene Bollinger are named as third in the Disinformation Dozen. The Tennessee couple, both devout Christians, have raked in millions through sales of supplements and documentary films and books questioning mainstream medicine, particularly chemotherapy treatment for cancer and vaccines.

'Have you had enough of the fake pandemic yet?' asks one 'example violation' post quoted in the report.

They also asked their followers to join them at a rally in Washington, D. C. on 6 January 2021, writing: 'Our internet is finally back up here in Nashville after the Christmas Day bombing. They will stop at nothing to steal this election and America. Be assured they will not win. Ty and I will be in DC on

Jan 6 speaking. We hope you will be there with us! #StopTheSteal #MAGA #Trump2020.' Although they clearly backed Donald Trump's baseless claim that he was cheated out of a re-election, there was no evidence that the Bollingers were in any way involved in that day's storming of the Capitol building.

Osteopath Sherri Tenpenny, an anti-vaxxer and ardent opponent of mask mandates, was number four on the list. On 23 June 2020, she was said to have tweeted: 'The #MaskAgenda has nothing to do with health and everything to do with control & suppressing your #immunesystem. The longer you wear one, the more unhealthy you become.'

Number five was Rizza Islam, whose anti-vaccine posts were allegedly aiming 'to spread vaccine hesitancy amongst African Americans'.

Rashid Buttar, another osteopath at number six, claimed COVID vaccines cause infertility and that COVID tests contained living organisms, according to the CCDH report.

Mercola's partner and founder of Health Nut News, Erin Elizabeth, is number seven followed by Sayer Ji, who runs another alternative anti-vax health site, GreenMedInfo.com, at number eight. One 'example violation' posted by Ji reads: 'The FLU has decided to identify as COVID-19 and we should all respect and support its decision.'

Ji's partner, Kelly Brogan, a practitioner of 'holistic psychiatry', is at number nine and gynaecologist Christiane Northrup rounds out the top ten, followed by chiropractor Ben Tapper, who tweeted to his followers: 'There is a total lack of evidence that viruses can live outside the body. When the whole healing profession comprehends this simple fact, there will no longer be this fear of germs, nor the need for vaccines, disinfectants, or other harmful germicides.'

Twelfth and final member of the Disinformation Dozen was anti-vaxxer activist Kevin Jenkins who has claimed that black people are being targeted with the vaccinations.

All twelve have complained that the social media platforms are attempting to silence them. Some have had accounts suspended and shut down and posts accompanied with misinformation warnings. But, as you will read, a leading anti-disinformation campaigner insists that big tech hasn't gone far enough and claims governments around the world were caught napping by the 'Infodemic'.

It is the battlefield of the twenty-first century – the war for the truth.

CHAPTER 22:

PULLING BACK FROM THE EDGE
– November 2018

▼

Lee McIntyre is not your archetypal philosopher with his head in the clouds or buried in books; he likes to talk to actual people to understand the world around us. As a Research Fellow at the Center for Philosophy and History of Science at Boston University and an instructor in Ethics at Harvard Extension School, he focuses on finding truth in the human experience.

His challenge when deciding to write a book about science deniers was to understand the thinking of people who, when confronted by scientific truth, choose to reject it, ignoring the facts and sometimes simple common sense.

That research would come into sharp focus once COVID-19 provided conspiracy theorists and media outliers with the perfect opportunity they had been waiting for to outwit officialdom and find the kind of huge audience for their views they could only have dreamed of before the pandemic.

But this was November 2018, and the Philosophy professor

was venturing into one of the deepest conspiracy theory rabbit holes by attending the Flat Earth International Conference (FEIC) in Denver, Colorado, along with 600 hard core devotees.

He spent two days with these people who believe that the Earth is a disc with the 'mountains of Antarctica' forming a boundary around it to prevent us from falling off the edge; the first day listening to their speeches and 'evidence' and the second discussing their beliefs and trying to get a handle on how they could believe them.

Attending seminars with titles like 'Globebusters', 'Flat Earth with the Scientific Method', 'Flat Earth Activism', 'NASA and other Space Lies', '14+ Ways the Bible say Flat Earth' and 'Talking to your Family and Friends about Flat Earth', felt, says McIntyre, 'in some ways like spending two days on another planet'.

'The arguments were absurd, but intricate and not easily run to ground, especially if one buys into the Flat Earthers' insistence on first person proof,' he wrote in *Newsweek* magazine. 'And the social reinforcement that participants seemed to feel in finally being 'among their own' was palpable. Psychologists have long known that there is a social aspect to belief. FEIC 2018 was a lab experiment in peer pressure.'

He continued: 'Most of the presentations were designed to show that the 'scientific' evidence for a global Earth was flawed, and that their own 'evidence' for Flat Earth was solid. Virtually all of the standards of good empirical reasoning were violated. Cherry-picking evidence? Check. Fitting beliefs to ideology? Check. Confirmation bias? Check. How to convince anyone in this sort of environment? You don't convince someone who has already rejected thousands of years of scientific evidence by showing them more evidence. No matter what I presented, there was always some excuse: NASA had faked the pictures from space. Airline pilots were in on the conspiracy. Water can't adhere to a spinning ball.'

The weird thing is that the Flat Earth movement is growing. You may think that the wealth of scientific information on the internet would show the deniers how the spherical Earth rotates on its own axis once every twenty-four hours, but apparently the deniers prefer to use the web to find like-minded disbelievers who share their views that we are the victims of a historic hoax.

Nevertheless, the Flat Earthers remain very much in the minority. They understand they're regarded as crackpots; it's part of the appeal – an exclusive club beyond the understanding of regular folks. It's like they are in on this monumental secret that nobody else understands.

COVID-19 conspiracists represent a much bigger – and more urgent – problem. Believing you fall off the edge of the world can undoubtedly cause social issues and alienation among friends and family, and you may lose your job or even get forced out of your church if you can't keep your theories to yourself – but it's not going to kill you. Go ahead, charter a boat to find the abyss but be sure to book a return ticket.

Denying that COVID is real can be deadly. If you don't believe me, keep reading the next few chapters.

Lee McIntyre may not have convinced anyone at the conference that the Earth was round; they were too deep into the rabbit hole to listen to scientific reason. But he did talk to the attendees. And he listened. And he came away with the idea that's it's not just that they were misinformed, but distrustful. 'If they weren't distrustful,' he said, 'the misinformation problem could be solved overnight. But because they don't trust the scientists and because they don't trust all these people who they say have been lying to them, it's impossible to convince them unless they trust you.

'A lot of them came to Flat Earth after some sort of trauma in their life. Now some of these are just garden variety traumas that we've all lived through, but for a number of the Flat Earthers, it was 9/11 because they were conspiracy theorists in their heart and soul and when they saw 9/11, they thought, well, this obviously is a conspiracy, and the mainstream media isn't saying that it is so they're lying to us. What else are they lying about? More than one person said to me, if they could lie to us about 9/11, what else could they lie to us about? Well, that rabbit hole goes pretty deep. It was almost like a religious conversion for them. Like something out of *The Matrix* where one day they woke up, took the red pill, and realized that the rest of the world didn't know they were being lied to.

'That relates to COVID especially because so much of it was new but went on trust. These people didn't really understand the science of it and probably didn't even take the trouble of trying to understand it, but they just distrusted what they were told. You don't convince somebody by cramming facts down their throat if they don't already trust you.

'I don't think a lot of people understand how science works. They don't understand that science isn't about proof, that uncertainty plays a role, that scientists change their mind when they get new data. And so that was very confusing for the public.

'Seventy years of social psychology has taught us that belief is social,' said McIntyre. 'If their identity is at stake, if they don't feel important, if they've now found a community of other people who believe what they believe, it makes them feel important, that they're part of something. It's how people end up in cults, it's how people get recruited into extremist political movements. It's just brainwashing.'

The problem with misinformation during the COVID pandemic is that the conspiracy theorists were way ahead of the authorities. Governments and health experts never got ahead of the problem because they were so far behind. McIntyre is convinced that was no accident. The misleaders-in-chief pounced on the opportunity provided by the pandemic for their own ends, whether that was cash, influence, power or something else.

'Somebody is intentionally creating disinformation for the purpose of misleading other people,' he explained. 'And they're not only misleading them about the facts; they're misleading them about who to trust. That distrust is not organic, it is cultivated, and the result of the relentless polarization. It's the goal of the disinformers. We saw this with the cigarette companies in the 1950s, we saw this with the fossil fuel companies around climate change in the seventies, eighties, nineties, and up until today, and we see it with COVID as well. It's unimaginable to rational people, but there are people out there who are serving their own interests, sometimes financial, but sometimes political, or are ideological, who want an army of people to believe a falsehood because it serves their interests.

'So, you've got this interesting thing with the deniers. They're not anti-science, they don't distrust all science, just the areas where they've gotten the disinformation. And so COVID for me is fascinating because we all got to see COVID denial arise, just organically out of nothing, kind of like climate denial only on steroids. I mean, it happened just incredibly fast.'

McIntyre published a book in 2021 titled *How to Talk to a Science Denier* (MIT Press) and is researching a new work on the disinformation crisis to reflect the threat highlighted by the pandemic. He is also the author of *Post-Truth* (MIT Press, 2018).

'I feel this is true about COVID more than anything else, more than 9/11 or the moon landings or any conspiracy theories – all these deniers are ordinary people. They are distrustful, to the extent that they're not getting vaccinated. These are your next-door neighbours; you don't sense a controversial bone in their body, but they have this view that perhaps they're not even sharing very widely.

'There was an incredibly successful disinformation campaign around COVID because it was life and death stakes, immediate, everybody was nervous. Nobody wanted to make a mistake. They piggybacked on the anti-vax movement that was already pretty big and then they politicized it. It's appalling to imagine that somebody is whipping that up on purpose, but they are doing it for their own purposes.'

As a board member of the Cognitive Immunology Research Collaborative (CIRCE), a think tank of psychologists and phil-osophers, cognitive scientists and evolutionary bio-logists, behavioural economists and information epidemiologists work-ing to prevent 'epidemics of unreason,' McIntyre and Andy Norman, CIRCE's founder, have been talking to governments, health departments, WHO and other organisations to share advice on how best to combat disinformation.

It's not just political leaders who were left flat-footed by the deniers; big tech also got caught out.

'In my opinion, the social media platforms are making the problem worse because they're not recognizing that it's actually an information war and they're putting a weapon in the hands of the people who are slaughtering others with the false information,' continued McIntyre. 'The number one thing that they could do is to de-platform the liars.

'People say, "What about free speech?" But in a polluted information stream, the lie wins out. It's to get you not just to believe the falsehood, but to doubt the truth, to get them to say, "I'll just believe what the people in my party believe or people in my family or the people in my social group believe." Truth doesn't stand a chance, it's not even close. It's not an even fight so the social media companies need to start de-platforming the liars. The way that social media companies handle that is so ridiculous. They will take down the bot accounts or they'll go after individual messages. They need to go after the liars. They know who they are. I don't know why they haven't de-platformed all of them. I take a very hard line on this because right now the liars are just out there with a megaphone spreading the lie everywhere. And people absolutely believe it.'

In their leaflet, 'How to Spot COVID-19 Conspiracy Theories', four experts, Stephan Lewandowsky, chair of - psychology at the University of Bristol, John Cook, postdoctoral research fellow with the Monash Climate Change Communication Research Hub, Ullrich Ecker, associate professor of cognitive science at the University of Western Australia, and Sander van der Linden, director of the Cambridge Social Decision-Making Lab, University of Cambridge, outlined seven 'traits of con-spirational thinking' under the acronym CONSPIR to explain the phenomenon.

'The COVID-19 pandemic is a fertile breeding ground for conspiracy theories,' they wrote. 'When people suffer a loss of control or feel threatened, they become more vulnerable to believing conspiracies. For example, the Black Death in the fourteenth century inspired anti-Semitic hysteria and when cholera broke out in Russia in 1892, blame fell on doctors and crowds hunted down anybody in a white coat.

'How do we avoid being misled by baseless conspiracy theories? Conspiracy theories are identified by tell-tale thought patterns. Learning these patterns is key to inoculating ourselves and society against the corrosive influence of conspiracy theories.'

Using the abbreviation CONSPIR, here are some tell-tale signs detailed in the online pamphlet for spotting a conspiracy theory:

C – Contradictory: Conspiracy theorists can hold incoherent beliefs, for example, believing that Princess Diana was murdered but also believing that she faked her own death. The conspiracy theorist is so committed to disbelieving the 'official' account that it doesn't matter that their theory is contradictory.

O – Overriding Suspicion: Conspiratorial thinking involves overwhelming suspicion towards the official account. This extreme degree of suspicion prevents belief in anything that doesn't fit into the conspiracy theory.

N – Nefarious Intent: The motivations behind any presumed conspiracy are invariably assumed to be nefarious. We see this in conspiracies about climate change when people allege that routine data adjustments are actually NASA intentionally 'cooking the books'.

S – Something Must Be Wrong: Although conspiracy theorists may occasionally abandon specific ideas when they become untenable, those revisions don't change their overall conclusion that 'something must be wrong' and the official account is based on deception.

P – Persecuted Victim: Conspiracy theorists perceive and present themselves as the victim of organised persecution. At the same time, they see themselves as brave antagonists taking on the villainous conspirators.

I – Immune to Evidence: Conspiracy theories are inherently self-sealing – evidence that counters a theory is re-interpreted as originating from the conspiracy. The stronger the evidence against a conspiracy (e.g., investigations exonerate climate scientists from allegations of misconduct), the larger the conspiracy must be (e.g., the investigations into climate scientists were part of the conspiracy)!

R – Re-interpreting Randomness: The overriding suspicion found in conspiratorial thinking frequently results in the belief that nothing occurs by accident. Random events are re-interpreted as being caused by the conspiracy and woven into a broader, interconnected pattern.

'Exposing the CONSPIR tactics will help raise awareness of the ways conspiracy theories distort the facts and is key to building resilience and inoculating ourselves and others from being misled, especially when we are most vulnerable: in times of crises and uncertainty,' wrote the authors in the May 2020 paper.

Lewandowsky, Cook and Van der Linden are also associates of CIRCE. One key strategy CIRCE push is to get out in front of the lies and McIntyre credits President Joe Biden for using the tactic effectively while dealing with Putin's invasion of Ukraine. They call it 'pre-bunking'. In an article written with Norman, who is also the author of *Mental Immunity: Infectious Ideas, Mind-Parasites, and the Search for a Better Way to Think* (Harper Wave, 2021), they explain how the White House began warning as long ago as December 2021 that Moscow might start spreading fake news to justify an invasion. The following month they gave details of a false flag operation in which Russia would release staged video 'evidence' of Ukrainians supposedly committing human rights atrocities and when the footage was actually released it was quickly dismissed as propaganda and ridiculed.

'That's how you combat disinformation,' they wrote in the *Deseret News*.

Biden's spokeswoman, White House Press Secretary Jen Psaki, explained the reasoning, saying at the time: 'We've made a decision – a strategic decision – to call out disinformation when we see it. We are much more cognizant of the Russian disinformation machine than we were in 2014. Russia has a boundless capacity to misrepresent truth.'

McIntyre and Norman go on to spell out the dangers of doing nothing. 'Our brave new digital world gives bad actors unprecedented power to exploit vulnerable minds. Russian propagandists, domestic conspiracy theorists, demagogic politicians, cult leaders, peddlers of quack cures – our world is now teeming with people skilled at disrupting higher brain function. Scientists call it 'amygdala hijacking' – the use of fear to sow division, stoke resentments, win followings and manufacture cynicism ... Disinformation is insidious. Like biological weaponry, it releases infectious agents that spread corruption among the susceptible. With internet connectivity as a vector of transmission, the threat to our way of life is profound.'

They add: 'In the future, once people become more aware of the prevalence of disinformation and the power of pre-bunking, it will be possible to head off some of this nonsense before it starts, by making people more sceptical of what they see and hear and building up their mental immunity in advance.'

We've heard about the Disinformation Dozen and their reasons for pushing back against COVID. We kind of know that anyone who believes the Earth is flat is likely to believe some of the more outlandish conspiracy theories swirling around during the pandemic. But what about the Russians?

The reality is that they invaded the West many years ago with very few people even noticing. They have messed with elections, smeared public figures and torn countries apart from within by setting families and countrymen against each other by promoting political polarisation.

But Putin's biggest triumph was his stealth mission to spread lies and conflict over COVID-19.

CHAPTER 23:

RUSSIA AND PATIENT 060606
– 29 April 2020

▼

The article appeared online eight months before the US rolled out its first vaccination. The headline in the *Oriental Review* story read: 'Bill Gates, Vaccinations, Microchips, And Patent 060606' and it began by mocking conspiracy theories like reptilians running the US government and 'Coca-Cola using the blood of Christian babies to produce its soft drinks'.

Crazy stuff, eh! Who'd believe stories like that?

And then it drops a whopper of its own, claiming a patent filed by Microsoft to implant a chip into the body 'that monitors a person's daily physical activity in return for cryptocurrency. If conditions are met, then the person receives certain bonuses that can be spent on something,' it adds.

There is no mention of chips being implanted in the patent, but that doesn't seem to matter in the report, which continues: 'Microsoft's involvement is interesting. And why has the patent been given the code number 060606? Is it a coincidence or the deliberate choice of what is referred to in the Book of Revelation as the number of the beast?

'Bill Gates' name is constantly being mentioned these days in connection with his interests in pharmaceutical companies, vaccinations, and WHO funding. Although the globalist media try to highlight Bill Gates as a great philanthropist and protect him from attacks and criticism in every way possible, it is unlikely they'll be able to conceal a whole web of connections.'

Then the article shows its true conspiracy theory colours with a rant against the West.

'Theological interpretations of the patent number are probably best left to experts on religion, but it is clear that there are strong links between organisations and companies like the Rockefeller Foundation, Microsoft, the pharmaceutical lobby and the World Bank Group, not to mention secondary service providers,' it reads, continuing: 'They are trying to play the role of a supranational government by constantly focusing on the fact that, these days, national governments cannot cope with epidemics, illnesses, famines, etc. single-handed. But, as China has shown, they can. The West cannot and does not want to acknowledge this, however, largely because it does not want to share power. So, the globalist media will continue their information campaigns, where the blame will be placed anywhere but on the West. It is telling that right now, as additional information on the coronavirus has started to emerge, false stories on China's role in the epidemic have been stepped up and statistics manipulated.'

The Moscow-based outlet has fewer than twenty-five employees and reaches a relatively small audience, but this story offers a prime example of how Russia secretly spread disinformation that fed into the West's hunger for alternative narratives. Flawed as it is, the <u>Oriental Review</u>'s concocted claim about Bill Gates provided the basis for the most popular and widely spread conspiracy theory of the pandemic – that Gates hid microchips in COVID-19 vaccinations as part of a plot to control the world.

It was one of the great successes of Russia's foreign military intelligence agency, the GRU, in its online campaign to disrupt America's COVID policies – and a technique it would use again to try and manipulate world opinion in the wake of the invasion of Ukraine. The Russian military calls it 'information confrontation'.

The Kremlin effectively weaponises the Internet as a means of surreptitiously spreading propaganda in the guise of news. While the strategy went largely unnoticed by the public and the media, it wasn't a mystery to Western intelligence services. In a report on Russia published in July 2020, the House of Commons Intelligence and Security Committee called Russian influence in the country 'the new normal'. Perhaps that explained why they did so little to stop it!

It's not like it's a new phenomenon. The Russians have been planting the idea that US scientists were responsible for past epidemics, such as the flu and Ebola, for years. As long ago as the 1970s, according to the *New York Times*, Putin was working in foreign intelligence for the KGB at a time it conducted a highly successful campaign suggesting that the virus that caused AIDS was developed by the Pentagon to kill black Americans. By 1987, the fake stories had reportedly run in eighty countries and twenty-five different languages and negatively impacted America's diplomacy abroad, especially in Africa. Only after the Cold War, reports *The Times*, did the Kremlin confess the stories were manufactured.

As Putin rose to power in Moscow, the fake news propaganda became a key part of his clandestine foreign policy. A concocted story in 2014 that an Ebola patient had been flown from Liberia to Atlanta caused a brief panic until it was disproven and a bogus 2017 video claiming a scientist who helped discover the AIDS virus wanted to depopulate the Earth got nearly four million views. A 2018 study by researchers at the University of California, Los Angeles, found that faked stories about AIDS over the years had such an effect on African Americans that many decided against seeking medical treatment. Putin's disinformation propaganda targeting vaccines has coincided with a drop in the number of American children getting jabbed and a rise in measles.

The public's vulnerability to faked news was highlighted in a 2017 poll by Survation which showed that more than half of British users of social media admitted they didn't check the original source of online material before they shared or 'liked' it.

An August 2020 report from the Global Engagement Center at the US Department of State, 'Pillars of Russia's Disinformation and Propaganda Ecosystem', details how the Russian authorities created and amplified false narratives through official, proxy and unattributed communication networks. 'The Kremlin bears direct responsibility for cultivating these tactics and platforms as part of its approach to using information as a weapon,' the report says. 'It invests massively in its propaganda channels, its intelligence services and its proxies to conduct malicious cyber activity to support their disinformation efforts, and it leverages outlets that masquerade as news sites or research institutions to spread these false and misleading narratives.'

There's no single source of disinformation; instead, the Russians rely on 'varied and overlapping' messages and stories that work to reinforce one another even though they may involve different subjects. Concocted stories will be repeated as facts and multiplied through different outlets until they appear to be the truth. Four of the Russian outlets – Global Research, SouthFront, New Eastern Outlook and Strategic Culture Foundation – published one another's content on 141 occasions, a clear sign of collaboration.

'The media multiplier effect can, at times, create disinformation storms with potentially dangerous effects for those Russia perceives as adversaries at the international, national, and local level,' the report reads. 'In the past, Russia has leveraged this dynamic to shield itself from criticism for its involvement in malign activity. This approach also allows Russia to be opportunistic, such as with COVID-19, where it has used the global pandemic as a hook to push longstanding disinformation and propaganda narratives,' it adds.

To illustrate the Russian disinformation strategy, the State Department document follows a story trumpeting a false claim that the US started the pandemic by launching a bioweapon attack on China. Five of the seven proxy sites outed in the report promoted this theory in a total of thirty articles starting on 20 February 2020, just as the world was coming to terms with the scale of the crisis and there was still a lot of confusion over its origin.

New Eastern Outlook published the first story in Russian and English followed two days later on 22 February by an adapted version of the same story in NewsFront's Bulgarian language edition.

RT, Russia's state-controlled international news network that can attract as many as one million views per day for its YouTube videos, published a story headlined 'Coronavirus May Be a Product of US Biological Attack Aimed at Iran and China, IRGC chief claims' on 5 March and that same story was republished by Global Research on 6 March and then by the German edition of NewsFront on 9 March.

On 16 March, Global Research ran a story saying the US had used a bioweapon on Cuba and two days later it carried another report saying China believed the virus was a bioweapon. By 20 March, the story had evolved with NewsFront suggesting an American lab in Georgia was involved in creating COVID.

The report lists the most active proxy sites and describes them as:

The Strategic Culture Foundation: An online journal registered in Russia that is directed by Russia's Foreign Intelligence Service (SVR) and closely affiliated with the Russian Ministry of Foreign Affairs. One of its core tactics is to publish Western fringe thinkers and conspiracy theorists, giving them a broader platform, while trying to obscure the Russian origins of the journal. This tactic helps the site appear to be an organic voice within its target audience of Westerners.

New Eastern Outlook: A pseudo-academic publication of the Russian Academy of Science's Institute of Oriental Studies that promotes disinformation and propaganda focused primarily on the Middle East, Asia and Africa. It combines pro-Kremlin views of Russian academics with anti-US views of Western fringe voices and conspiracy theorists. New East-ern Outlook appears to want to benefit from the veneer of respectability offered by the Russian academics it features, while also obscuring its links to state-funded institutions. According to the report, an example of its COVID disinformation was a 28 February 2020 article that read: 'With high probability the virus was man-made in one or several bio-warfare laboratories of which the Pentagon and CIA have about 400 around the world ... But such high-security bio-labs also exist in Canada, the UK, Israel, and Japan. Western media also are silent about the fact that the virus is directed specifically at the Chinese race, meaning it targets specifically Chinese DNA. Almost all the deaths or infected people in the thirty-three countries and territories to which the virus spread, are of Chinese origin ... this is in whatever way you want to turn it, a bio-war against China.'

Global Research: A Canadian website that has become deeply enmeshed in Russia's broader disinformation and propaganda ecosystem. Its large roster of fringe authors and conspiracy theorists serves as a talent pool for Russian and Chinese websites. Its publications also provide a Western voice that other elements of the ecosystem can leverage to their advantage. Global Research made headlines on 12 March 2020 when China's Ministry of Foreign Affairs spokesman Zhgao Lijian posted two tweets linking to stories wrongly claiming that the US caused the COVID pandemic.

NewsFront: A Crimea-based disinformation and propaganda outlet with the self-proclaimed goal of providing an 'alternative source of information' for Western audiences. With reported ties to the Russian security services and Kremlin funding, it is particularly focused on supporting Russia-backed forces in Ukraine. NewsFront's manipulative tactics to boost reach led to a near total dismantling of its presence on social media in early 2020. Among the false narratives peddled by NewsFront, which claims to have offices in the UK, are the following:

• The United States created the coronavirus as a bioweapon, tested deadly viruses on humans in Ukraine and China, developed bacteriological weapons specifically aimed at certain ethnic groups, intentionally infected US-based migrants with COVID-19 and transported the virus to China.

• Cooperation with Europe is a catastrophe for Ukraine. Ukraine has become a colony of the IMF and George Soros and its president is a CIA puppet. Ukraine cannot control the coronavirus, as more than 1,500 Ukrainian soldiers in Donbas are infected with COVID-19. Nazis are patrolling Kyiv's streets, and a Ukrainian army veteran drove a truck into demonstrators in Minneapolis.

• The EU is dead, it cannot handle the COVID-19 pandemic, and has abandoned Ukraine. The EU is inflaming the war in Donbas and is attempting to destabilise Belarus.

• NATO did not provide any COVID-19 assistance to Spain, does not care about Montenegro and spreads the coronavirus in the EU.

• Bill Gates is linked to the COVID-19 outbreak and uses the pandemic to implant microchips 'in whole of humanity [sic]'. COVID-19 vaccines are a fraud spearheaded by Gates and Big Pharma.

SouthFront: A multilingual online disinformation site registered in Russia that focuses on military and security issues. With flashy infographics, maps and videos, SouthFront combines Kremlin talking points with detailed knowledge of military systems and ongoing conflicts. It attempts to appeal to military enthusiasts, veterans and conspiracy theorists, all while going to great lengths to hide its connections to Russia. The report says examples of SouthFront's COVID disinformation include:

• 'Phenomena of Coronavirus Crisis': 'Financial circles and governments are using the coronavirus to achieve own financial and political goals.'

• COVID-19 – The Fight for a Cure: One Gigantic Western Pharma Rip-Off: 'The real question is – are vaccines – or a vaccine – even necessary? Maybe – maybe not. The production of vaccines is pushed for profit motives and for an important political agenda for a New World Order.'

• The Coronavirus COVID-19 Pandemic: The Real Danger is 'Agenda ID2020': 'There is not the slightest trace of a pandemic ... If indeed force-vaccination will happen, another bonanza for Big Pharma, people really don't know what type of cocktail will be put into the vaccine, maybe a slow killer, that acts-up only in a few years – or a disease that hits only the next generation – or a brain debilitating agent, or a gene that renders women infertile ... all is possible – always with the aim of full population control and population reduction.'

• USA Plan: Militarized Control of Population. The 'National COVID-19 Testing Action Plan': 'The 'pandemic response body' would above all have the task of controlling the population with military-like techniques, through digital tracking and identification systems, in work and study places, in residential areas, in public places and when travelling. Systems of this type – the Rockefeller Foundation recalls – are made by Apple, Google and Facebook.'

• Finally! EU Blames 'Kremlin Disinformation' for Coronavirus Crisis: 'EU bureaucrats and affiliated propaganda bodies are doing something that all has expected a long time ago – blaming Russia for the crisis over the outbreak of coronavirus.'

• COVID-19 Crisis in Russia: lockdown Craziness and Opposition Provocations: 'Summing up, it becomes obvious that anti-government Western-backed forces are trying to use the COVID-19 crisis to destabilize the situation in Russia.'

Geopolitica.ru: Serves as a platform for Russian ultra-nationalists to spread disinformation and propaganda targeting Western and other audiences. Inspired by the Eurasianist ideology of the Russian philosopher and Eurasian imperialist Alexander

Dugin, Geopolitica.ru views itself as caught in a perpetual information war against the Western ideals of democracy and liberalism. The website's cooperation with other outlets in Russia's disinformation and propaganda ecosystem broadens the reach of its messaging, which seeks to destabilise and weaken Western institutions. The report lists its fake COVID stories as follows (they include the same Bill Gates story that appeared in *Oriental Review*):

• 'Bill Gates, vaccinations, microchips, and patent 060606' promotes a conspiracy theory attacking Bill Gates and the Micro-soft Corporation for an alleged plot to control humans by inserting microchips into their bodies. The article suggests a possible link between the Microsoft's patent number WO/2020/060606 and the 'number of the beast' from the 'Book of Revelation'.

• 'Russia and the coronavirus' asserts that Western media spread disinformation about the number of COVID-19 related deaths in Russia and suggests that 'one of the reasons why COVID-19 mortality rates are very low in Russia is that many Russians do not get flu vaccinations imported from the West'.

• 'New Malthusianism and the misanthrope dynasties' falsely claims that the US government and Bill Gates aim to reduce the world's population, also alleging that Gates helped create the Zika virus.

• 'The Coronavirus and hybrid warfare' speculates that COVID-19 is a part of a US strategy 'aimed at undermining the economic growth of both China and other countries' or a 'plot by transnational capital against Donald Trump on the eve of the presidential election'.

• 'Former Putin's aide: Coronavirus is the US biological weapon' quotes Sergey Glazyev, a member of Katehon's supervisory board member, and a former advisor to President Putin, as claiming that the COVID-19 virus is a US biological weapon targeting 'mostly people of the yellow race' and blaming Great Britain for provoking Hitler at the outbreak of World War Two.

• 'Pandemic in the service of globalization'– blames the EU/Atlanticist/Globalist powers for intentionally inflating the threat posed by the COVID-19 pandemic to "deepen the automation of society" for the benefit of "corporate capitalism" and the "world government".

'The Italian government at the time of the coronavirus' argues that the coronavirus crisis in Italy demonstrates that the values of the Germany-dominated EU are not the values of the Italian people, and that the EU's economic recipes have been lethal for Italy.

'Pandemic and the survival policy: the horizons of a new form of dictatorship' claims that COVID-19-related restrictive measures in Western societies amount to 'total surveillance of the population' and will 'gradually become permanent', spelling the 'end of liberal democracies and the establishments [sic] of dictatorships throughout the world'. This looming 'dictatorship' is described as potentially 'harsher than Nazi and Soviet concentration camps'.

Katehon: A Moscow-based quasi-think-tank that is a proliferator of virulent anti-Western disinformation and propaganda via its website, which is active in five languages. It is led by individuals with clear links to the Russian state and the Russian intelligence services. Within Russia's broader disinformation and propaganda ecosystem, Katehon plays the role of providing supposedly independent, analytical material aimed largely at European audiences, with content allegedly dedicated to 'the creation and defense of a secure, democratic and just international system'. Among the conspiracy theories on Katehon's website, according to the report, are:

• The British House of Commons considers the coronavirus a blessing.

• The coronavirus is a French-made virus transferred by the Americans.

• The coronavirus is an ethnic biological weapon.

• The coronavirus is a US tool to disrupt Chinese production.

• The United States owns the coronavirus and its cure.

• The original source of the coronavirus is a US military biological warfare laboratory.

The United States created coronavirus in 2015.

• Science doubts the effectiveness of vaccines.

Interestingly, a big majority of the tweets sharing these Russian proxy articles came from the UK. The State Department report claimed the top ten locations for the accounts tweeting these stories between 1 April and 30 June 2020, were:

UK (16 per cent)

Russia (9 per cent)

Canada (7 per cent)

Japan (6 per cent)

France (5 per cent)

Spain (4 per cent)

Chile (4 per cent)

Venezuela (4 per cent)

Germany (3 per cent)

Australia (3 per cent)

In that same time period, the most used hashtags in these tweets were:

#COVID19 (4,358 tweets)

#coronavirus (2,265 tweets)

#us (949 tweets)

#billgates (867 tweets)

#china (718 tweets)

The most shared article – tweeted more than 15,000 times – appeared on the Strategic Culture Foundation website and claimed a German official leaked a report dismissing COVID-19 as a 'global false alarm'. It was denounced by the German government, who said a disgruntled employee used an official letterhead to support his own views.

Lea Gabrielle, head of the Global Engagement Center, told the US Senate Foreign Relations Subcommittee on 5 March 2020, that the Russians were using the pandemic to 'take advantage of a health crisis where people are terrified'.

'The Kremlin often swamps the media environment with a tsunami of lies,' she said. 'Outside of Russia, the Kremlin seeks to weaken its adversaries by manipulating the information environment in nefarious ways, polarizing domestic political conversations, and attempting to destroy the public's faith in good governance, independent media, and democratic principles.'

She continued: 'The Russian government directs and supports these propaganda activities globally, but especially targets and seeks to nurture the most extreme or divisive elements of society in the United States, Europe, and other regions in which they operate. We see in many Western Hemisphere countries the same tactics used by the Kremlin and its proxies.

'These include cyber-enabled disinformation operations; propaganda campaigns that seek to rewrite history; coordinated social media swarms that inflame existing fault lines of societies, and an array of other actions that fall within the scope of their malign information operations. We have seen these tactics time and time again, from right here at home to the streets of the capital cities of our allies.

'The Kremlin does this to hide its own role in tragic events, such as the downing of Malaysia Airlines Flight 17 (MH17) and the nerve-agent poisoning of UK citizens in Salisbury, England. They do this in support of the murderous Assad regime by smearing credible voices on the ground in Syria with false information. They do this to prop up the regime of Nicolás Maduro in Venezuela and suppress legitimate democratic voices, and they do this in an attempt to weaken solidarity within NATO.'

In a 3 March 2022 press release, the US Department of the Treasury named Oriental Review, Strategic Culture Foundation, New Eastern Outlook, Geopolitica, NewsFront and SouthFront as outlets 'propagating Russian intelligence services-directed content' and announced its Office of Foreign Assets Control was targeting them, along with a number of Russian oligarchs and their families, for economic sanctions.

On 31 March, Britain's Foreign Secretary Liz Truss also announced sanctions against some key figures behind Putin's propaganda machine, including heads of RT and the state news agency Sputnik and seven people linked with the Strategic Culture Foundation.

It took the war in Ukraine for Britain and the US to finally take strong action against the Kremlin's fake news network, but as we will learn, it was way too late to stop the out-of-control narrative on COVID. Too much damage had already been done.

I can attest to the Russians' attempt to 'legitimise' their fake news machine. During the latter period of my twenty-five years in New York and Los Angeles as a journalist covering the United States for the *Daily Mail*, the London *Evening Standard*, *Newsweek* and other publications, I received several calls from producers at RT asking me to work as a correspondent for them in America. I declined, as did colleagues working as foreign correspondents, knowing that any stories, however apparently innocuous, would likely be twisted to suit Moscow's own particular narrative.

While there is clearly evidence that the Russians have manipulated the truth delivered to foreign audiences, the obvious question is why do they spend so much time and effort making up stories? It is certainly cheap; the costs are marginal when compared to a superpower defence budget. And it works. The Wild West nature of online news offers unlimited opportunities to skip around the editing and fact-checking required of legitimate news outlets. In some cases, especially involving false stories denigrating the Pfizer and other Western COVID vaccines, the purpose was commercial, hoping to boost Russia's own Sputnik V at the expense of its competitors.

'The emphasis on denigrating Pfizer is likely due to its status as the first vaccine besides Sputnik V to see mass use, resulting in a greater potential threat to Sputnik's market dominance,' said a report by the Alliance for Securing Democracy, part of a US think tank.

But Lee McIntyre, Research Fellow at Boston University's Center for Philosophy and History of Science, sees the Kremlin's intentions as more ideological. It wants to tear down the very fabric of America's defining democracy.

'In my view, the goal here is for Russia to undermine Western institutions that are meant to promote truth,' he explained. 'In just the same way that they interfered with the 2016 election, in order to undermine democracy, they desire to interfere with Western science, because it is another pillar of American society. And why would they do this for the COVID vaccines in particular? Money and prestige. The Russians had the Sputnik V vaccine and wanted it to become the world standard, for sale in Africa and Asia, to bring them money and status. Putin sees the 'vaccine wars' as another space race ... hence the name 'Sputnik' for their vaccine! He's not subtle.'

Not surprisingly, Russia denies the existence of a disinformation campaign. 'It's nonsense,' Kremlin spokesman Dmitry Peskov told the *Wall Street Journal*. 'Russian special services have nothing to do with any criticism against vaccines. If we treat every negative publication against the Sputnik V vaccine as a result of efforts by American special services, then we will go crazy because we see it every day, every hour and in every Anglo-Saxon media.'

The great irony is that the Kremlin's disinformation offensive against the West, and the US in particular, was so successful that it backfired in Russia. They did such a good job in spreading anti-vax propaganda that they couldn't persuade Russians to get jabbed – even Putin hesitated and waited about seven months to take it.

One July 2020 opinion poll put the percentage of Russians who had doubts about the vaccine at 90 per cent, although that figure later dropped to half of the country. A year later, another poll suggested that 62 per cent of Russians were still prepared to go unvaccinated.

Despite being the first vaccine developed, Russia's prized Sputnik V was a flop internationally where it had been promoted as an alternative to Western shots. People had read the stories; they didn't trust it.

CHAPTER 24:

A FEMALE RAPPER AND A DIFFICULT CASE OF SWOLLEN BALLS
– 13 September 2021

▼

Nicki Minaj clearly thought it was important to give her 24.8 million followers on Twitter a heads-up.

'My cousin in Trinidad won't get the vaccine cuz his friend got it & became impotent,' she tweeted on 13 September 2021. 'His testicles became swollen. His friend was weeks away from getting married, now the girl called off the wedding. So just pray on it & make sure you're comfortable with ur decision, not bullied,' she continued.

Now she certainly got a global backlash with everyone from UK Chief Medical Officer Chris Whitty to Trinidad and Tobago's health minister telling the rapper in more diplomatic terms that she was tweeting a load of bollocks. Prime Minister Boris Johnson was forced to admit during a Downing Street press briefing that he was 'not as familiar with the works of Nicki Minaj as I probably should be' and the White House even offered her a call with one of President Joe Biden's doctors to set her straight.

'There's no evidence that it happens, nor is there any mechanistic reason to imagine that it would happen,' insisted Dr Anthony Fauci, America's leading expert on infectious diseases.

Whitty thought the Trinidadian-born star should be 'ashamed'.

But none of that prevented Minaj's tweet from racking up 146,700 likes and 24,600 retweets. An earlier tweet she posted that same night, explaining why she wasn't going to the star-studded Met Gala in New York garnered another 72,200 likes.

'They want you to get vaccinated for the Met,' she tweeted. 'If I get vaccinated it won't for the Met. It'll be once I feel I've done enough research. I'm working on that now. In the meantime my loves, be safe. Wear the mask with 2 strings that grips your head & face. Not that loose one.'

Medical experts lined up to insist that vaccinations posed no threat to male or female fertility, but the rumour persisted. You can bet there were plenty of people who would believe Minaj over Whitty and Fauci. After all, the singer was doing her own research!

As with most things regarding COVID, there was a much more serious side to consider. From the earliest days of the pandemic, stories have circulated about the dangers the jabs represent to pregnant mothers. As a result, a considerable percentage of expectant mums have elected against being vaccinated and some have paid with their lives.

The medical profession was insistent that the various COVID-19 vaccines were entirely safe and caused neither fertility issues nor problems at any stage of pregnancy. Health officials were adamant that vaccines do not contain live coronavirus and cannot infect a pregnant woman nor her unborn baby in the womb. Data from the UK Health Security Agency appears to bear this out. It showed that vaccinated women who gave birth between January and October in 2021 had a very similar low risk of stillbirth, low birthweight and premature birth compared to women who were not vaccinated in pregnancy.

At the same time, the risk of mothers-to-be falling seriously ill with COVID appeared much higher if they were unvaccinated. Out of 235 pregnant women admitted to intensive care with COVID between January and September 2021, none of them had received the recommended two doses of vaccine.

The NHS statistics suggest that the vaccine doesn't harm expectant women or their children. They show that:

• The stillbirth rate for vaccinated women who gave birth was approximately 3.6 per 1,000, a similar rate for women who were not vaccinated in pregnancy (3.9 per 1,000).

• The proportion of vaccinated women giving birth to babies with low birthweight (5.01 per cent) was lower than the proportion for women who were not vaccinated in pregnancy (5.33 per cent).

• The proportion of premature births was 5.97 per cent for vaccinated women, similar to the 5.88 per cent in women who were not vaccinated in pregnancy.

'All the evidence is showing that having the vaccine is safe for you and your baby and is the best way to protect you both against this potentially serious, and deadly, virus. Hundreds of thousands of pregnant women across the USA, the UK and elsewhere have had the vaccine with no harms to them or their baby reported,' said Dr Mary Ross-Davie, Director for Professional Midwifery at the Royal College of Midwives. 'I urge pregnant women who have not yet been jabbed to go to trusted sources for their information about the vaccination such as the RCM or NHS websites, midwives and doctors, and not to be influenced by the mass of incorrect misinformation swirling around the internet and social media.

'It is also particularly important that we work to increase levels of vaccination in pregnant women in communities where the uptake is low. A concerted effort is needed to engage with these women, and to support them with advice and information about the vaccine, about its safety and about its benefits,' she added.

I come from the generation with mothers who were told it was fine to take a drug called Thalidomide for morning sickness, only to discover too late that it killed their babies or left them with severe deformities in their limbs, so it is entirely understandable to me that pregnant women should be hesitant to risk their child's health, let alone their own, with a newly developed vaccine.

Perhaps the heartbreaking stories of new mothers who contracted COVID offer a more persuasive argument than any doctor or government official could ever manage.

Three unvaccinated women who gave birth while sick with COVID shared their stories in a video made by the NHS and the UK government to try and persuade unvaxxed mothers-to-be to get the jab.

'So, I was week thirty,' said the first of the three new mothers, named only as Christina. 'I go into hospital because I thought I was going to deliver a baby. They actually wake me up and told me that I have COVID. My symptoms started to arise and they were quite bad. They were starting to worsen. They had to do CT scans to see if I was having a preliminary embolism because of the clotting. I did ask them if COVID would've affected her (baby), they said unlikely, but because it affected her foetal growth restriction, she is more mostly likely to have maybe developmental issues in the future. So, we don't know. And when you don't know, you have that anxiety continuously.'

The second woman, Joanne, said: 'I'm getting COVID. It was quite a scary time, especially when they're telling me that they think the COVID did affect my placenta around the cord to the baby, so she was lacking oxygen. I've totally changed my mind from not wanting the vaccine to straight away wanting the vaccine. For the baby's sake if anything, I had to get the vaccine.'

'So I was about thirty-two to thirty-three weeks' pregnant at that stage when we both got COVID following the birth of my son,' said Tanviha, the third new mother featured in the film. 'He was taken straight to ICU in Burnley, and I continued to deteriorate.

'I was still in ICU, and I was still receiving CPAP then. I had a conversation with one of the consultants in ICU that it would be best to ventilate me just to give my lungs a rest. But you know, my family lived through every day. They lived through the phone calls and being told that I may not survive – potentially having to say goodbye to me on a ventilator. As a family, it was such a big part of our lives, more for my husband and my family.'

Professor Asma Khalil, a Professor in Obstetrics and Maternal Foetal Medicine, goes on to say: 'Over the last few months, we have data from a very large number of pregnant women, more than 300,000 pregnant women from the United States, more than 90,000 pregnant women in the UK. We know that the vaccine is effective. We know that it does not increase the risk of miscarriage. It does not increase the risk of still births. It does not make the women go into premature birth. And therefore, the advice is clear. The best way for a pregnant woman to protect herself and her baby is to get a COVID vaccine.'

'We know that it's so safe for pregnant women to have it,'

adds Christina. 'I really strongly advise that they should because I don't want them to experience what I went through. I unfortunately couldn't get it at the time, but if I could have, I, I definitely would have.'

Houston, Texas, mother-of-two Diana Crouch spent five months in hospital with COVID after deciding not to get vaccinated because she was afraid it would harm her unborn baby. Her husband, Chris, told ABC 13: 'The reason, obviously, for her was because she didn't think it would be good to get a vaccine while she was pregnant. The doctors said all of this could have been avoided if she was vaccinated. We'll never know at this point.'

Diana suffered three strokes on the same day and a heart attack, as well as seizures, and gave birth at just thirty-one weeks but was expected to make a full recovery following the birth of her son, Cameron – who was named after a medical director at the hospital where she was treated.

'I didn't really have any concerns about it,' Diana told the *Houston Chronicle*. 'What could possibly go wrong if you eat healthy and you've had kids before? You don't really think much of it besides it being another flu.

'After everything that I went through, all the drugs they put in my body, that should have been the least of my worries,' Diana said of the vaccine. 'I was on so many drugs, very strong drugs, and so much was done to my body, I just don't think the vaccine could have been that bad for me.

'We'll never know if getting the vaccine would have made a difference, but it could have made a difference,' she added.

Sadly, some unvaccinated mothers were not so lucky. Their COVID symptoms were so bad they couldn't overcome them.

Saiqa Parveen, thirty-seven, from Birmingham, decided to

wait until after her baby was born before getting the jab. But she was taken to hospital with breathing difficulties in September 2021 and was put on a ventilator to help her breathe. Her baby was born by Caesarean section when she was eight months' pregnant, but Saiqa died on 1 November after suffering further complications, including sepsis, without ever getting the chance to hold her newborn, fifth child. Her brother, Qayoum Mughal, told the BBC that his sister received a letter offering her the vaccine, but she told her family: 'It's too late now, when I've had my baby I will get my vaccine. But she didn't get the chance.

'If she had the vaccine, she might have had a chance of surviving,' he added. 'For the sake of God and the sake of your loved ones, please get vaccinated.'

Natalie Forshaw, thirty, from Manchester, decided against getting vaccinated before giving birth to her son on 3 November 2021, because she was worried about its possible effects on the baby. She had an emergency Caesarean after testing positive for COVID and appeared to be recovering when she collapsed and was rushed to intensive care at Manchester Royal Infirmary and passed away on the Boxing Day.

In the United States, a twenty-seven-year-old unvaccinated mother from Texas fell sick with COVID while pregnant with her sixth child. Doctors delivered Crystal Hernandez's baby by emergency C-section in January 2022 and she appeared to be on the mend, but her health suddenly deteriorated, according to ABC 13, and she died in mid-January. Her husband, Rio, was reported as saying that the couple hadn't been vaccinated because 'it all happened so fast, and it was being pushed on us very fast – she was pregnant and so she had some concerns.'

Stephanie Baker, thirty-one, from North Carolina died from

COVID three days after giving birth to twins in January 2022. One of her newborns also died after an emergency Caesarean carried out after her babies showed signs of distress from a lack of oxygen.

Her mother, Debbie, told *Newsweek* her 'beautiful, inside and out' daughter didn't get jabbed because she was worried it would affect her babies. 'She just thought, "I gotta protect them and I don't want anything to hurt them", and I respect that [because] she loved her children,' she said. 'But I was always thinking "what if" and just praying, "Please don't let her get COVID, please let her make it through this pregnancy and be healthy." And she chose not to, and I respected that,' Debbie added. The heartbroken mother urged pregnant women to get vaccinated. 'We would never push anything on anyone, but it's devastating to go through this, and I wouldn't want anyone else to go through such pain,' she said.

Whether they believed the horror stories about vaccinations or simply worried about the possible side effects on their unborn children, unvaccinated pregnant women appeared to make up a worryingly high proportion of people worst affected by COVID.

Between July and September 2021, according to NHS England, unjabbed pregnant women made up nearly one-fifth of the most critically ill COVID-19 patients.

Expectant mums who hadn't had a first vaccine dose accounted for 17 per cent of COVID patients treated with an emergency lung bypass machine in England. They also made up around a third of all women aged between sixteen and forty-nine being treated in intensive care with extracorporeal membrane oxygenation, the highest level of life support after a ventilator that functions as a heart and lungs outside the body. This statistic had risen from 6 per cent at the outset of the pandemic in March 2020.

Dr Nikki Kanani, NHS England's head of primary care, said being pregnant puts extra strain on the woman's heart and lungs. If the expectant mum gets COVID, that 'lays on pressure on an already pressurised system inside a pregnant woman, and that's why almost 20 per cent of people with coronavirus who are having extra support on critical care are pregnant women who are unvaccinated,' she told the BBC.

Stories of very human tragedies are sprinkled through the pandemic, often with links to conspiracy theories.

Samantha Wendell, from Kentucky, decided to hold off on her vaccination before her wedding after hearing claims that the jab caused infertility. The twenty-nine-year-old and her fiancé, Austin Eskew, hoped to have three or four children and he said his wife-to-be 'just kind of panicked'.

Instead of attending Samantha's wedding in 2021, Eskew and their families were at her funeral at the same church after she lost a six-week battle with COVID.

'Misinformation killed her,' Samantha's cousin, Maria Vibandor Hayes, thirty-nine, told NBC News. 'If we can save more lives and families' lives, then this is the gift that she left for us to deliver.'

Her family said that before she was put on a ventilator, Samantha asked to be vaccinated. 'It wasn't going to do any good at that point, obviously. It just weighs heavy on my heart that this could have easily been avoided,' said her mother.

Another young mother, Dezi Scopesi, twenty-three, from Utah, died after delaying her vaccinations because she was concerned it could affect breastfeeding her baby. Dezi contracted COVID along with her husband and baby, but she never recovered.

Kelly Ernby, a rising star in the Republican Party in Orange

County, California, was an outspoken opponent of vaccine mandates and when she passed away from COVID at the age of forty-six, her death became a lightning rod of controversy.

In August 2021, she had written on Facebook: 'The vaccine is not the cure to COVID, and mandates won't work.'

'There's nothing that matters more than our freedoms right now,' she told a Republican rally.

After her death, the *Los Angeles Times* reported an explosion of comments online 'blaming her for her own death'.

'She did this to herself,' said one post. 'Congratulations on winning your very own Darwin award,' read another.

Friends said they received hundreds of upsetting messages on social media condemning her anti-vax views.

Communities, neighbourhoods, families and marriages: they have all been torn apart over conflicting views about what the pandemic is, how it came about, and, perhaps most importantly, how it should be controlled.

It doesn't seem to make any difference when a fervent anti-vaxxer dies from COVID or when a blushing bride-to-be worries that a jab might mess up her wedding plans and ends up gasping for air in a hospital bed; the vaccination doubts have a habit of sneaking into the national psyche.

And it's not always as obvious as someone becoming convinced that Bill Gates wants to know how many times you are going to the bathroom or that snakes are being slithered into your bloodstream.

Often, people just don't believe it is going to happen to them.

The nearly 3,000 people who died on 9/11 woke up that sunny morning with a multitude of thoughts and moods, worrying about work and relationships and all those daily details that make up a life. But even in their worst nightmares, they never thought they would be the innocent victims in a faraway war most had only seen on the television news. COVID is much closer to home, and the majority of us, vaccinated and unvaccinated, socialists and conservatives, will come through it relatively unscathed. We go on with our lives, as best we can. We don't expect to get it and, if we do, we don't think it will kill us.

There is always the exception, of course – one man in Bristol tested positive for COVID forty-three times.

But more than 6.2 million people around the world have died during the pandemic, 173,000 of them in the UK.

And every one of them has a story.

CHAPTER 25:

THE IVY LEAGUE 'CONSPIRACY THEORY'

– 2–4 October 2020

▼

The blueprint to get a grip on COVID was direct and simple. The young and healthy are absolved of any lockdown mandates and free to go about their business while the old and vulnerable are hidden away. If you are young and unhealthy, well, you might have to just take your chances with the rest of the herd.

You may think it's the plot of a Hollywood blockbuster like *The Matrix 5* or *Blade Runner 7* or the latest deep state conspiracy from David Icke. The more cynical may believe it's Vladimir Putin's latest ploy to deceive the West with a sinister suggestion that the old and the sick are dispensable.

But what if I was to tell you this was a plan proposed by three scientists, all at the very tops of their fields, from Harvard, Oxford and Stanford universities? Dr Martin Kulldorff is a professor of medicine at Harvard University, a biostatistician and epidemiologist with expertise in detecting and monitoring infectious disease outbreaks and vaccine safety evaluations; Oxford University Professor Dr Sunetra Gupta is an epidemiologist with expertise in immunology, vaccine development and mathematical modelling of infectious diseases and Dr Jay Bhattacharya, professor at Stanford University Medical School, a physician, epidemiologist, health economist and public health policy expert focusing on infectious diseases and vulnerable populations.

This is how they describe themselves on a website laying out their plan to save the world and asking for signatures to a declaration supporting their 'focused protection' approach.

Among the co-signers from the medical world from the UK are Dr Anthony J Brookes, professor of genetics, University of Leicester, Dr David Livermore, microbiologist, infectious disease epidemiologist and professor, University of East Anglia, Dr Helen Colhoun, professor of medical informatics and epidemiology, and a public health physician, Dr Paul McKeigue, physician, disease modeller and professor of epidemiology and public health, and Dr Simon Wood, biostatistician and professor, all from the University of Edinburgh, Dr Matthew Ratcliffe, professor of philosophy, specialising in philosophy of mental health, University of York, Dr Stephen Bremner, professor of medical statistics, University of Sussex, Dr Lisa White, professor of modelling and epidemiology, Oxford University, Dr Mike Hulme, professor of human geography, University of Cambridge, Dr Yaz Gulnur Muradoglu, professor of finance, director of the Behavioural Finance Working Group, Queen Mary University of London, Dr Angus Dalgleish, oncologist, infectious disease expert and professor, St. George's Hospital Medical School, University of London, Dr Ellen Townsend, professor of psychology, head of the Self-Harm Research Group, University of Nottingham,

Dr Gabriela Gomes, mathematician studying infectious disease epidemiology, professor, University of Strathclyde, Dr Karol Sikora, physician, oncologist and professor of medicine at the University of Buckingham, and Dr Mario Recker, malaria researcher and associate professor, University of Exeter.

Also on the list of co-signers is a Nobel Prize winner, Dr Michael Levitt, a biophysicist and professor of structural biology, Stanford University (recipient of the 2013 Nobel Prize in Chemistry) and Michael Jackson (research fellow, School of Biological Sciences, at the University of Canterbury in New Zealand, not the late entertainer!).

Anyone is going to agree that's a heavyweight academic crew. They certainly wouldn't describe themselves as conspiracy theorists. They clearly believed enough in the proposals being put forward by Kulldorff, Gupta and Bhattacharya to add their names to the declaration along with more than 928,000 others, including 15,840 medical and public health scientists and 46,893 medical practitioners.

Some pranksters added fake names like Dr Johnny Bananas, Prof. Spon'Ge'Bob SQ.UarePants, Dr Neal Ferguson, Prof. Ware Thamask, and Dr Person Fakename but they made up less than 1 per cent of the total and most have been removed.

The mission statement was written by the Ivy League trio between 2 and 4 October 2020, at the American Institute for Economic Research, located in Great Barrington, Massachusetts and was subsequently titled, The Great Barrington Declaration. It's relatively short, so I include it in full:

The Great Barrington Declaration – As infectious disease epidemiologists and public health scientists we have grave concerns about the damaging physical and mental health impacts of the prevailing COVID-19 policies, and recommend an approach we call Focused Protection.

Coming from both the left and right, and around the world, we have devoted our careers to protecting people. Current lockdown policies are producing devastating effects on short and long-term public health. The results (to name a few) include lower childhood vaccination rates, worsening cardiovascular disease outcomes, fewer cancer screenings and deteriorating mental health – leading to greater excess mortality in years to come, with the working class and younger members of society carrying the heaviest burden. Keeping students out of school is a grave injustice.

Keeping these measures in place until a vaccine is available will cause irreparable damage, with the underprivileged disproportionately harmed.

Fortunately, our understanding of the virus is growing. We know that vulnerability to death from COVID-19 is more than a thousand-fold higher in the old and infirm than the young. Indeed, for children, COVID-19 is less dangerous than many other harms, including influenza.

As immunity builds in the population, the risk of infection to all – including the vulnerable – falls. We know that all populations will eventually reach herd immunity – i.e. the point at which the rate of new infections is stable – and that this can be assisted by (but is not dependent upon) a vaccine. Our goal should therefore be to minimise mortality and social harm until we reach herd immunity.

The most compassionate approach that balances the risks and benefits of reaching herd immunity, is to allow those who are at minimal risk of death to live their lives normally to build up immunity to the virus through natural infection, while better protecting those who are at highest risk. We call this Focused Protection.

Adopting measures to protect the vulnerable should be the central aim of public health responses to COVID-19. By way of example, nursing homes should use staff with acquired immunity and perform frequent testing of other staff and all visitors. Staff rotation should be minimised. Retired people living at home should have groceries and other essentials delivered to their home. When possible, they should meet family members outside rather than inside. A comprehensive and detailed list of measures, including approaches to multi-generational households, can be implemented, and is well within the scope and capability of public health professionals.

Those who are not vulnerable should immediately be allowed to resume life as normal. Simple hygiene measures, such as hand washing and staying home when sick should be practiced by everyone to reduce the herd immunity threshold. Schools and universities should be open for in-person teaching. Extracurricular activities, such as sports, should be resumed. Young low-risk adults should work normally, rather than from home. Restaurants and other businesses should open. Arts, music, sport and other cultural activities should resume. People who are more at risk may participate if they wish, while society as a whole enjoys the protection conferred upon the vulnerable by those who have built up herd immunity.

The response, I suggest, was nothing like as mind-blowing as the authors and their supporters may have hoped. What reaction there was appears to have been negative with Gregg Gonsalves, an epidemiologist at Yale University, one of the most outspoken detractors, arguing that lockdowns were necessary to cut infection levels and suggesting in a 5 October 2020 Twitter thread that 'these herd immunity strategies are about culling the herd of the sick and disabled. It's grotesque.'

In a string of tweets, Gonsalves dissects The Great Barrington Declaration, writing:

For a start, we are in agreement that the pandemic has created indirect harms for many beyond the direct effects of infection with the virus itself. These cannot be ignored and need to be addressed head-on.

BUT rather than address the real indirect effects this pandemic has caused, they suggest that the best way to deal with the matter is to increase the DIRECT causes of harm instead.

They suggest that we should focus on protecting the elderly and vulnerable, and let everyone else go about their business, get infected to build herd immunity in the population. That's the main gist of it.

Let's start with the elderly. Most of the elderly in the US are NOT in nursing/care homes. Yes, we should protect those in nursing homes, where we have seen much of the mortality in the US, but the track record even there is terrible thus far.

Now, a large chunk of the elderly in the US live with family or are alone or with their similarly elderly spouses – that is they are integrated into the community. How do you pull these older people to safety? What's the plan?

If you're going to turbocharge community spread,

as everyone else at 'low-risk' goes about their business, I want the plan for my eighty-six-year-old mother to be more than theoretical. They do NOT have one.

Now let's deal with the vulnerable. This is where their strategy goes even further off the rails. CLOSE to 50 per cent of ALL Americans have underlying conditions that predispose them to severe #COVID19 outcomes...

So, we have now arguably the majority of the population – the elderly, chronically ill and disabled – who are going to have to be sequestered while the young and fit go about their business, catching the disease, building up herd immunity.

And for these three, #COVID-19 isn't something to worry about if you're young and healthy, if you're young and not so healthy, well, you're out of luck in their brave new world...

I get it. We're all tired. This pandemic sucks. The measures we've had to take are terrible too. But beware of the answers you want to hear: it's OK, if you're not at high-risk, get back out there, help build herd immunity, it's scientific!

William Hanage, a professor of epidemiology at Harvard, also took issue with the declaration, telling the *Guardian*: 'After pointing out, correctly, the indirect damage caused by the pandemic, they respond that the answer is to increase the direct damage caused by it.'

Shocked at the personal attacks and the way their plan had been portrayed in some parts of the media and scientific community, Jay Bhattacharya, Sunetra Gupta and Martin Kulldorff doubled down on their declaration with an additional explanation on 25 November 2020, suggesting it was a 'middle ground between lockdowns and "Let it Rip"':

This may surprise some readers given the unfortunate caricature of the Declaration, where some media outlets and scientists have falsely characterized it as a 'herd immunity strategy' that aims to maximize infections among the young or as a laissez-faire approach to let the virus rip through society. On the contrary, we believe that everyone should take basic precautions to avoid spreading the disease and that no one should intentionally expose themselves to COVID-19 infection. Since zero COVID is impossible, herd immunity is the endpoint of this epidemic regardless of whether we choose lockdowns or focused protection to address it.

The premise of the Declaration rests on two scientific facts. First, while anyone can get infected, there is more than a thousand-fold difference in COVID-19 mortality between the oldest and youngest. Children have lower mortality from COVID-19 than from the annual influenza. For people under the age of seventy, the infection survival rate is 99.95 per cent. We now have good evidence on the relative risk posed by the incidence of chronic conditions, so we know that among common conditions, age is the single most important risk factor. For instance, a sixty-five-year-old obese individual has about the same COVID-19 mortality risk conditional upon infection as a seventy-year-old non-obese individual.

Second, the harms of the lockdown are manifold and devastating, including plummeting childhood vaccination rates, worse cardiovascular disease outcomes, less cancer screening, and deteriorating mental health, to name a few. The social isolation induced by lockdown has led to a sharp rise in opioid and drug-related overdoses, similar to the 'deaths of despair' that occurred in the wake of the 2008 Great Recession. Social isolation of the elderly has contributed to a sharp rise in dementia-related deaths around the country. For children, the cessation of in-person schooling since the spring has led to 'catastrophic' learning losses, with severe projected adverse consequences for affected students' life spans. According to a CDC estimate, one in four young adults seriously considered suicide this past June. Among 25- to 44-year-olds, the CDC reports a 26 per cent increase in excess all-cause mortality relative to past years, though fewer than 5 per cent of 2020 deaths have been due to COVID-19.

The harms of lockdown are unequally distributed. Economists have found that only 37 per cent of jobs in the US can be performed wholly online, and high-paying jobs are overrepresented among that set. By declaring janitors, store clerks, meat packers, postal workers, and other blue-collar workers as 'essential' workers in most states, regardless of whether they qualify as high COVID mortality risk, the lockdowns have failed to shield the vulnerable in these occupations. The economic dislocation from the lockdowns has increased the number of households where young adults who have lost their jobs co-reside with vulnerable older parents, which may increase the risk of COVID-related death. In addition, school closures have contributed to shortages of nurses and other medical personnel who stay home to care for their children rather than work. Very clearly, exposing people to the medical and psychological harms from the lockdowns is ethically fraught.

The two main planks of focused protection and The Great Barrington Declaration follow logically from these two facts. For older people, COVID-19 is a deadly disease that should be met with overwhelming resources aimed at protecting them wherever they are, whether in nursing homes, at their own home, in the workplace, or in multi-generational homes. For the non-vulnerable, who face far greater harm from the lockdowns than they do from COVID-19 infection risk, the lockdowns should be lifted and – for those who so decide – normal life resumed.

So, what happened with The Great Barrington Declaration and the work of all these great minds? The answer is, not a lot. The mainstream media had become so wary of conspiracy theories during the pandemic that the merest whiff of a controversial theory sent it running for the hills. Running down fake news became a full-time job during the Trump presidency. When it came to COVID, journalists and producers preferred to ignore outlier ideas altogether if possible unless they originated from the White House or Downing Street or became impossible to avoid through the manipulative megaphone of Fox News.

The Great Barrington Declaration may have been built on a sturdy foundation of doctorates and academic prizes and reinforced with a barrage of citations, but it smelled of a conspiracy theory. Talk of the old and the sick being culled, however sensationalist, makes editors and politicians nervous. It can even lose elections.

Toby Young in *The Spectator* made no secret of his support for the declaration; he urged readers to sign it and included the website, insisting they should 'ignore the censors and the smear merchants'.

'The three scientists who created it aren't outliers or cranks, but professors at Oxford, Harvard and Stanford,' he wrote in his 17 October 2020 magazine column.

'And since its launch, the declaration has been signed by tens of thousands of epidemiologists and public health scientists, including a Nobel Prize winner.

'So why haven't you heard of it? The short answer is there's been a well-orchestrated attempt to suppress and discredit it. I searched for it on Google last Saturday and the top link was to an article in an obscure left-wing magazine claiming the petition was the work of a 'climate science denial network' funded by a right-wing billionaire. The top video link was to a *Channel 4 News* report in which Devi Sridhar, a public health advisor to the Scottish government, denounced the declaration as not 'scientific'. A bit rich considering Devi's PhD is in Social Anthropology, whereas Sunetra Gupta, one of the petition's authors, is a global expert on infectious diseases. In the first ten pages of Google search results, not one took me to the actual declaration'.

He continued:

'It is hard to find any mention of it on Reddit, the world's best-known discussion website. The two most popular subreddits devoted to the virus – r/COVID19 and r/Coronavirus – have excised all references to it, with the moderators of the latter denouncing it as 'spam'. A similar line has been taken by nearly all left-leaning newspapers. the *Guardian* ran an article on the declaration last

Saturday, but only to flag up that its more than 400,000 signatories included a handful of dubious-sounding 'experts', such as 'Dr Johnny Bananas' and 'Prof Cominic Dummings'. Hardly surprising, given that lockdown zealots have been openly encouraging their followers on social media to sign up with fake names.'

Young said it got even worse when the BBC asked Professor Gupta, one of the declaration authors, not to mention it during an interview about lockdowns.

The speed with which vaccines were rolled out in the West played a part in undermining the idea of focused protection and herd immunity. Vaccines superseded lockdowns and the conversation quickly faded into the background. Interviewed in August 2021, Professor Bhattacharya was adamant that he and his colleagues were vindicated, saying: 'We've been vindicated. The lockdowns were the single biggest mistake in public health history. I don't see how anyone can look at lockdown and say, 'That was successful policy.' We've had lockdowns in country after country after country. Would you call lockdown a success in the UK?'

But he admitted to being 'shocked' at the backlash against the declaration, telling UnHerd's Freddie Sayers: 'I was naive, I have spent my career in academia. I've not spent my career in politics ... I didn't know that people would then use *ad hominem* attacks against me ... I expected more serious engagement by serious people.'

Just because people question the official narrative, even if their arguments don't ultimately hold up, doesn't necessarily mean they are conspiracy theorists. As long as their views are not offensive and don't have the potential to cause harm, then they deserve to be heard, whether you are a scaffolder or a Nobel Prize winner. More on this later.

But how does that work if you're a physician? What about that trust between a doctor and their patient that has been the foundation of our health services since Imhotep, the first physician to the pharaohs? The doctor told me so it must be true, the saying goes.

You don't need to wear masks – it's not the law.

COVID wards in UK hospitals are empty.

COVID cases are really 'normal, healthy people'.

The pandemic ended in June 2020.

Flu is a bigger killer than COVID-19.

Under-45s have more chance of being hit by lightning than dying of COVID.

A positive PCR test doesn't mean that someone is infected or infectious...

These are some of the claims made by an organisation called the World Doctors Alliance, featuring a group of current and retired doctors from seven countries, including NHS surgeon Dr Mohammad Adil and Dr Dolores Cahill, who got her PHD in Immunology and Biotechnology from Dublin City University. The group currently has 146,000 subscribers on Telegram and its Facebook following grew from 4,000 in March 2020 to more than 460,000 by June 2021, according to the *Guardian*. Videos posted by the group on Facebook have been viewed more than 21.1 million times. There is an appetite out there for this stuff.

In one 2020 WDA video, viewed hundreds of thousands of times, Elke de Klerk, a GP from Holland, denies there was a pandemic, but says COVID-19 is a 'normal flu virus' and that the crisis was 'created by false positive PCR tests'.

De Klerk maintained that 89–94 per cent of PCR tests were false positives.

Fact-checking for the Associated Press, another doctor and Harvard expert insisted: 'Many can be late positives meaning the RNA is still there, but the viable virus has been cleared. So, these people may not be contagious anymore. But the result is accurate – the PCR is finding SARS2 RNA.'

If doctors and some of the world's leading academics can't agree on the correct course of action, or even whether the pandemic was real, how do we stand a chance?

CHAPTER 26:

THE SILVER BULLET HORSE DEWORMER

– 13 November 2020

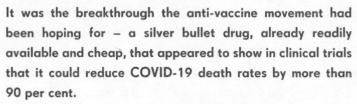

It was the breakthrough the anti-vaccine movement had been hoping for – a silver bullet drug, already readily available and cheap, that appeared to show in clinical trials that it could reduce COVID-19 death rates by more than 90 per cent.

Ivermectin may have been developed chiefly as an anti-wormer for horses and cattle and used to treat head lice, parasitic worms and scabies in humans, but if the 600-patient study proved correct, the drug had the potential to turn the coronavirus from a stealthy assassin into little more than an annoying pest.

The premise was simple. The researchers said they found 400 people with COVID-19, and they had another 200 healthy people who all agreed to take part in the study. The volunteers were randomly given Ivermectin or a placebo and the result, they claimed, was that those lucky people who got the Ivermectin were 90 per cent less likely to die than those who struck out with the placebo. It was a game-changer.

The initial research was still a preprint and did not have the weight of the scientific community with the necessary checks and peer reviews, but it still generated considerable excitement on 13 November 2020, when six researchers from two Egyptian universities uploaded their paper, 'Efficacy and Safety of Ivermectin for Treatment and prophylaxis of COVID-19 Pandemic' on to the Research Square preprint server.

Although it hadn't passed through the scientific safeguards required of a paper that has passed peer review or been published in a scientific journal, it was nevertheless cited in as many as thirty other studies, including some in prominent journals, according to the GRFTR debunker website.

But it wasn't only scientists and academics who took note. Doctors used the results of the study to justify using Ivermectin for their COVID patients. Suddenly, there was a run on the drug in pharmacies and demand was so great that farmers were complaining that animal feed stores were out of dewormers and prices were skyrocketing. According to the US Centers for Disease Control and Prevention, prescriptions for the drug soared from 3,600 a week before the pandemic to 88,000 a week.

Key to the study's overnight impact was its size – the largest of its kind to date – and its claims that not only did it reduce the number of deaths and the time in hospital spent by patients, but also helped prevent people from getting the disease.

Ivermectin was discussed on the floor of US Congress, with one doctor describing it as a 'wonder drug' and telling a Senate committee, 'If you take it, you will not get sick.' Such was the groundswell of interest in Ivermectin that it was promoted a number of times in the House of Commons.

According to Hansard, former Conservative Party Leader Sir Iain Duncan Smith said during Prime Minister's Questions on 20 October 2020: 'There is a lot of talk at the moment about the two antivirals that have now arrived, Remdesivir and Ivermectin. Given the Government's objective of driving down the infection rate, and given that the average age of death at the moment is 82.4, should we not make those antivirals much more widely available at the earliest opportunity, through GPs and every other doctor, in order to get them to people to reduce the likelihood of their going into hospital and dying?'

In a COVID debate on 12 January 2021, another senior Tory MP John Redwood said: 'What about Ivermectin, which some doctors in other countries say can also achieve good results and reduce the death rate? It would be useful to know what progress is being made with the UK tests and whether that might ever be a recommended treatment, because the more treatments we can have to cut the death rate the better.'

At another PM's Questions on 27 January 2021, David Davis, a one-time Conservative chairman, seemed to be referencing the study when he asked: 'Some Ivermectin studies have shown 75 per cent reductions in death rates. What scope is there to act quickly this winter – this winter, not next winter – to enhance our primary care level to protect populations and hospitals?'

Crossbench peer Lord Bilimoria, the British Indian business-man who built the Cobra beer brand, also told the House of Lords on 20 April 2021: 'Another aspect that not many people talk about is this: could the Government put the same focus, energy and investment as they did into the vaccination programme into turbocharging, at speed, the research and trials for authorising repurposed therapeutics and drugs? Dexamethasone was the first, but there are quite a few others, including Ivermectin, which could possibly cure over 80 per cent of COVID cases. Such drugs, if proven, would literally be game-changers against this wretched virus.'

For nearly six months, the Ivermectin paper went unchallenged, offering what appeared to be a viable alternative to vaccines, preventing infection as well as heading off its worst symptoms. Six countries including India and Peru officially promoted it as a COVID drug. One public health expert in Peru estimated that fourteen out of every fifteen COVID patients admitted into hospital had been taking Ivermectin.

The big problem was that this great Hail Mary clinical trial that was supposed to save us all from COVID was later withdrawn amid a scandal, with the researchers accused of fabricating data and plagiarising their introduction following an investigation by London medical student Jack Lawrence.

With a simple Google check, Lawrence easily confirmed that most of the study's introduction had been lifted from different sources without attribution. He told the *Guardian* that the authors had used a thesaurus to change some of the words, adding: 'Humorously, this led to them changing "severe acute respiratory syndrome" to "extreme intense respiratory syndrome" on one occasion.'

Then he started to notice that the numbers in the paper didn't add up. One anomaly appeared to be that one-third of the patients in the study who died from COVID were already dead before the researchers started looking for volunteers to take part and about a quarter of the patients were already in hospital with COVID before the trial began.

'The authors claimed to have done the study only on eighteen to eighty-year olds, but at least three patients in the dataset were under eighteen,' Lawrence told the *Guardian*. 'The authors claimed they conducted the study between 8th June and 20th September 2020, however most of the patients who died were admitted into hospital and died before the 8th June, according to the raw data. The data was also terribly formatted and includes one patient who left hospital on the non-existent date of 31/06/2020.'

He continued: 'In their paper, the authors claim that four out of 100 patients died in their standard treatment group for mild and moderate COVID-19. According to the original data, the number was 0, the same as the Ivermectin treatment group. In their Ivermectin treatment group for severe COVID-19, the authors claim two patients died, but the number in their raw data is four.'

Lawrence concluded his report: 'Thousands of highly educated scientists, doctors, pharmacists, and at least four major medicines regulators missed a fraud so apparent that it might as well have come with a flashing neon sign. That this all happened amid an ongoing global health crisis of epic proportions is all the more terrifying. For those reading this article, its findings may serve as a wake-up call. For those who died after taking a medication now shown to be even more lacking in positive evidence, it's too late. Science has corrected, but at what cost?'

In a 15 July 2021 Medium article, Gideon Meyerowitz-Katz, an epidemiologist at the University of Wollongong who was alerted to the discrepancies in the study by Lawrence, claimed that, if true, the allegations regarding the Ivermectin paper could be 'the most consequential medical fraud ever committed.'

He continues:

'It appears that one of the pivotal, key trials of Ivermectin in humans may be an elaborate work of scientific fraud. It's hard to know if the study even happened. If true, this may mean that Ivermectin has absolutely no benefit for COVID-19, and tens of millions of people worldwide have been scammed.

'It has been more than six months since this study was put online,' he concluded.

'By all signs, the results of this research have been used to treat thousands, or perhaps even millions, of people across the world. And yet until now no one noticed that most of the introduction is plagiarised?

'The scientific community, we noble defenders of truth, have well and truly cocked it up ... I don't know for sure that this study is fraudulent, and perhaps we never will. But we do know that no one should ever have used it as evidence for anything regardless. We will have to reckon with the fact that a truly woeful piece of research, which may turn out to be fraud, was put online and used to drive treatment to millions of people around the world. And no one noticed until it was far, far too late.'

Research Square later withdrew the preprint, saying: 'Due to an expression of concern communicated directly to our staff, these concerns are now under formal investigation.'

But the Egyptian study wasn't the only one boasting world-changing results – or facing questions over its authenticity. A 2020 trial in Argentina went one better by claiming Ivermectin prevented 100 per cent of COVID-19 infections, but critics pointed out 'inconsistencies' in a report by BuzzFeed.

A BBC investigation found that more than one-third of twenty-six Ivermectin trials for use on COVID patients show 'serious errors or signs of potential fraud' and 'none of the rest show convincing evidence of ivermectin's effectiveness'.

A group of scientists decided to work together and investigate Ivermectin trials after Lawrence uncovered the shortcomings of the Egyptian study. The team, which included Gideon Meyerowitz-Katz, Dr James Heathers, Dr Nick Brown and Dr Kyle Sheldrick, found there may have been faked evidence in five of the twenty-six trials and red flags in another five, with data and percentages not adding up.

They suggested that many of the trials showed that the sicker people tended to be in placebo groups while those with good measurements were those taking the Ivermectin doses, effectively rigging the results.

The health authorities in the UK, the United States and the European Union have all warned against the use of Ivermectin, saying there is no evidence to back claims that it is effective against COVID. America's Food and Drug Administration went so far as to tweet: 'You are not a horse. You are not a cow. Seriously, y'all. Stop it,' and link it to an article titled 'Why You Should Not Use Ivermectin to Treat or Prevent COVID-19'.

'There's a lot of misinformation around, and you may have heard that it's okay to take large doses of Ivermectin. It is *not* okay,' the story reads, adding: 'Even the levels of Ivermectin for approved human uses can interact with other medications, like blood-thinners. You can also overdose on Ivermectin, which can cause nausea, vomiting, diarrhoea, hypotension (low blood pressure), allergic reactions (itching and hives), dizziness, ataxia (problems with balance), seizures, coma and even death.'

None of this has stopped supporters of Ivermectin spreading the word that it works and there are still clinical trials under way to see if it does have any benefits for COVID patients, one of them at Oxford University as part of a British government study to improve recoveries outside hospitals. A small pilot programme showed taking Ivermectin early could ease the symptoms suffered by someone with a mild dose of the disease.

A Japanese study also showed Ivermectin showed an 'anti-viral' effect against Omicron, the COVID variant.

While governments and the mainstream media remained united against the use of Ivermectin, right-wing pundits in the US like Fox News' Tucker Carlson and Laura Ingraham were pushing it to their audiences and podcaster Joe Rogan was taking it on his show after contracting COVID and claiming he felt great.

TikTok was rife with pro-Ivermectin videos. 'I've said it before and I'll say it again in my videos – online, human consumption, 12 mg. Just take a lot of water with it. It worked great for my husband,' a woman says in a TikTok video watched by more than one million people. Other pro-Ivermectin videos had as many as five or six million views before they were taken down.

What would be the point in putting a dodgy clinical trial out there? Do the Ivermectin crew so desperately need some verified science to hang their views upon? Probably not, right. Is it possible that the apparently shoddy methodology of some of the studies have taken away from the positives the drug may offer to the COVID medicine cabinet? Maybe.

There are many passionate voices out there who are adamant that Ivermectin is the answer and that they are not conspiracy theorists.

Dr Pierre Kory, an American doctor who gave evidence about Ivermectin to the US Senate on 8 December 2021, has continued to be an advocate for use of the drug, insisting it has been thoroughly tested and that it works. A video of his Senate testimony went viral and was taken down after eight million views on one channel.

In a YouTube video streamed live on 5 May 2021, Kory claimed Ivermectin 'works in prevention, it works early, and it works late, it saves lives'.

Far from dismissing the clinical trials, he calls them 'gold standard' and is unapologetic about his advocacy for the drug. 'I have never heard of a medicine sitting on top of as formidable an evidence base as Ivermectin sits without a worldwide recommendation. It is absolutely unconscionable what is happening with Ivermectin,' he says.

'From the prevention trials, taking it regularly you can protect yourself from COVID. On average, on all the protocols, that's an 85 per cent protection rate ... If you take it nearly every week it's nearly perfect. If you take it weekly, you don't get sick and so it's incredible its prevention properties.

'If you look at mortality, there's not a lot of medicines that reduce mortality rates by the minimum of 68 per cent for late treatment and 80 per cent in early treatments,' says Kory, founder of the Front Line COVID-19 Critical Care Alliance (FLCCC).

'Trial after trial after trial ... It's very rare that you study a medicine with a dozen or more trials and you see all the treatment effects lining up on one side. It's almost a beautiful sight and yet they get attacked everywhere. The trials are small, they're poorly designed ... You hear nothing but insane arguments trying to argue against this truth. It's right there in the eye of the beholder.'

Dr Tess Lawrie, from Bath, formed the British Ivermectin Recommendation Development Group (BIRD) after watching Kory's Senate testimony and becoming convinced the drug should be at the forefront of attempts to cut the mortality and morbidity associated with COVID.

'Our evidence shows that Ivermectin is effective, safe and very cheap,' Lawrie said in a video message 'to the public' that was watched 17,000 times. 'We should be using it for both prevention and treatment of COVID. However, governments and health organisations are ignoring the evidence and there is a mountain of it. I think this is because they are heavily invested in novel treatments. So, I am asking you, please, take responsibility for your health, educate yourselves, inform your friends and family and, most of all, speak to your doctors. Help us spread the word, help us save lives.'

A good start would be to find some agreement on the veracity of the studies on Ivermectin. The Oxford University research could be key. Perhaps then we can agree on whether it can help us. Currently it's not approved for the treatment of COVID in the UK, but can be prescribed by doctors 'under their own responsibility'.

Some other so-called 'cures' are a little easier to judge.

Garlic was always good to ward off vampires or over-eager suitors, so I am told, but it's not much better than a carrot or a parsnip for protecting you from COVID. Clearly one woman in China didn't get the message – she needed hospital treatment for a badly inflamed throat after eating 1.5kg of raw garlic.

A social media post suggesting that drinking water every fifteen minutes flushes out the coronavirus was shared over 250,000 times, but experts say the only effect will be repeated trips to the toilet.

A fake UNICEF post claimed that drinking hot water and sunbathing for at least two hours kills the virus and eating ice cream attracts it. Another rumour did the rounds saying COVID could be destroyed with a hairdryer. In the end, UNICEF was forced to warn people about the misinformation, saying: 'A recent erroneous online message ... purporting to be a UNICEF communication appears to indicate that avoiding ice cream and other cold foods can help prevent the onset of the disease. This is, of course, wholly untrue.'

American televangelist Jim Bakker was sued for selling a

liquid silver solution on his streaming TV show as a cure for COVID-19. Bakker and his Missouri church agreed to pay restitution to people who bought the 'Silver Solution' – silver particles suspended in a liquid that supposedly build the immune system. Experts say the skin can turn blue if too much is taken, and the silver settles in the body tissue.

America's Food and Drug Administration and Federal Trade Commission also sent out warning letters to tea manufacturers claiming a cuppa could cure COVID, makers of essential oil who said their products could soothe away the virus, and makers of vitamin C and D vitamins.

Claiming that products like essential oils or vitamins can cure COVID are obviously false, as good as they may be for you in other ways, but it's still worth pointing out that building the immune system (terrain) with immune boosters is just good sense. And using essential oils like lavender which are anti-viral would help to strengthen a person's defences.

In the 1800s, Louis Pasteur paved the way for antibiotics and vaccines with his findings that germs or microorganisms are the cause of most diseases, while his friend, psychologist Claude Bernard, was insistent that the body's terrain was more important than the pathogens that infected it. He argued that his terrain theory explained why some people get sick while others do not despite being exposed to the same germs.

A story that Pasteur recanted on his deathbed to agree that a body's 'soil' was more important is said by some to be apocryphal. Nevertheless, with modern medicine still working in 'catastrophic mode' nearly 200 years later, it is surprising that public advice on beating COVID still ignores the importance of strengthening the immune system to stave off the virus.

And then there's the black market. Apparently, you could

snaffle an Oxford-AstraZeneca vaccine ($500), Johnson & Johnson and Sputnik V ($600 each), and Sinopharm ($750) from the dark web if you knew how to get there. From the same corner of the internet, you could buy a drug vaccine against COVID – a mix of amphetamines, cocaine and nicotine – for $300.

In India, claims that vegetarians were immune from COVID caused the hashtag '#NoMeat_NoCoronaVirus' to trend on Twitter and there was even a false rumour that curries helped keep the virus at bay, especially the hotter dishes.

CHAPTER 27:

SAVING THE WORLD AND CUTTING DOWN ON OAT CAPPUCCINOS
– April 2022

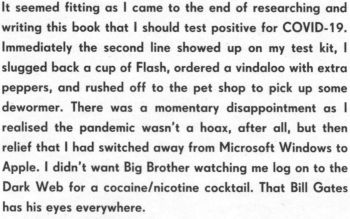

It seemed fitting as I came to the end of researching and writing this book that I should test positive for COVID-19. Immediately the second line showed up on my test kit, I slugged back a cup of Flash, ordered a vindaloo with extra peppers, and rushed off to the pet shop to pick up some dewormer. There was a momentary disappointment as I realised the pandemic wasn't a hoax, after all, but then relief that I had switched away from Microsoft Windows to Apple. I didn't want Big Brother watching me log on to the Dark Web for a cocaine/nicotine cocktail. That Bill Gates has his eyes everywhere.

Okay, so that didn't happen. For the record, I am vaccinated – two doses (Oxford-AstraZeneca) and a booster (Pfizer), so my experience with the virus was relatively mild. My self-prescribed treatment was to up the Vitamin C and D3, go easy on the oat cappuccinos for a couple of days and go for a run to try and shake it off.

My experience with a virus that has blighted so many lives is probably the norm – a nasty cough, razor blades in the throat for a few days and a thumping headache – but I understand that so many people have had it so much worse. The statistics, if you choose to believe them, certainly suggest that vaccination makes the symptoms easier to handle.

When I set out to write this book, my intention was not to judge the so-called conspiracy theorists and certainly not to demean those who follow them, but to put them into context as best I could and allow the readers to make up their own minds. I am not a doctor, a scientist and certainly not a politician and I do not believe my opinion to be any more valuable than anybody else's.

I do, however, believe that conspiracy theories in the era of COVID are different from those that came before. They have real-time consequences. It is not an exaggeration to say that they can kill. Read some of those stories of families hearing their loved ones on their deathbeds saying they wished they had been vaccinated and tell me they don't move you. Mothers losing daughters, babies losing mothers, families being wiped out. That's real; nobody is making up these stories.

You can attend Flat Earth conventions, argue until you are blue in the face that the Moon landings were faked or that JFK was assassinated by the Mafia and life will go on the same. With 9/11, as important as it is to get to the truth about what happened, it is not going to change the fact that nearly 3,000 people were killed. Even the most despicable conspiracy theory of all, the absurd and incredibly hurtful claim that the Sandy Hook school shooting that left twenty children aged between six and seven dead, was a hoax perpetrated by opponents of the second Amendment, is in the past. Nothing is going to change what happened, as much as we wish it could.

In the pandemic, people are listening to dissenting voices on YouTube and on social media and they are making decisions that will affect their lives and those of others based on those opinions. Can you blame people if they believe the opinions of distinguished academics or doctors?

Other than extreme cases – I'm sorry, I don't believe COVID is a giant hoax or vaccines contain mini-octopi creatures and, much as I distrust the disproportionately wealthy, I can't see Bill Gates as some nerdy Dr Evil – I have tried to leave the reader to make up their own minds about the various conspiracy theories discussed in this book.

It seems clear to me that boundaries are necessary. In the past, it was much easier for the gatekeepers to control the kind of material covered by the mainstream press and TV. As much as they were politically biased, newspapers generally took care to edit out the crazies and the print and broadcast media were both regulated; whether that be enough or too much is debatable. You can complain that newspapers don't care about getting a ticking-off from regulators, but I know from the experience of working for national newspapers for many years that they most certainly do. A complaint about a story, especially a formal complaint, is a black mark for any editor or reporter involved if they are proved to be true and not easily forgiven.

But conspiracy theories in the pandemic are an online phenomenon. If there is to be new regulation it must focus on internet content and it must be independent. How can Facebook or Twitter regulate itself when the very people they must rule over are driving traffic – and money – to their platforms?

The Office of Communications (Ofcom) and the Independent Press Standards Organisation (IPSO) carry weight watching over the broadcast and print media in the UK, although neither are completely independent.

IPSO, formed in 2014, is the successor to the Press Complaints Commission (PCC) that was scrapped in the wake of the News International hacking scandal. In its 2020/21 *The COVID Report*, IPSO asserted that the print media did a good job covering the crisis. Chairman Lord Faulks QC wrote that 'the press has played a vital role during the COVID-19 pandemic, informing the public of critical public health information and scrutinising the response to this unprecedented global health crisis. It is clearer now than ever how essential it is for the public to be able to turn to trusted, accountable sources of news at such testing moments.'

He said that of 30,000 complaints IPSO received about the print media in 2020, only about 10 per cent – or about 1,270 articles – were about COVID.

'This represents a vanishingly small slice of the coverage that COVID attracted throughout the UK press, from the time that the scale of the story started to emerge in February 2020 – including countless reports, graphs, 'explainers', comments and investigations,' he added. 'I have no doubt that journalism published by IPSO-regulated titles over the last eighteen months saved lives, in the UK and around the world.'

IPSO CEO Charlotte Dewar summed up the 'underlying challenge that we faced: how to protect the right to challenge, to provoke, to scrutinise as a free press should, at a time when lives were at stake, and information was incomplete at best. While in some cases we found examples where individual pieces of journalism had fallen short of the standards we expected, this dialogue between science and journalism was crucial to improving scientific understanding and informing the public.'

One example of how complaints about a 'fake' photograph was investigated illustrates how conspiracy theories can rage over the simplest of things. IPSO received twenty-two complaints that a snap showing people packed on to Brighton beach at a time social distancing rules were in force published on the front page of the *Daily Express* was staged. The complainants claimed the photo was taken the previous summer and that cranes shown in the background had since been removed. The *Express* was able to easily prove when the photo was taken from the metadata and the complaints were rejected. But that didn't stop the story from gaining a life of its own online. *Notting Hill* actor Hugh Grant, a founder of the Fleet Street watchdog group Hacked Off, was among the thousands of people retweeting the photo and claims it was faked.

The original tweet, from a Brighton resident, read, '@daily_Express just wondering why you're using a photo of Brighton seafront from last year? Those cranes are no longer there, couldn't be that you're working with the govt to put the blame on the public not them for this could it?'

Before it was deleted, it was retweeted 576 times and totted up 1,345 likes, according to the *Press Gazette*.

Rob Shepherd, another Brighton local, followed up with a post that was retweeted 2,800 times that read: 'This is a photo of Brighton and Hove seafront. I walk or run on this patch every day; I take my daughter for her exercise here every day. I have NEVER seen it looking like this during lockdown. This must be a photo from before lockdown. If so, it's disgracefully dishonest.'

Jon Mills, photo editor at South West News, the agency that filed the picture, answered Shepherd by tweeting the data from the camera and writing: 'Here is the original photo with its embedded metadata. Before we put it on our newswire we verified the camera date, interviewed the photographer and cross checked with other pictures taken around the same time. While we don't get everything right, we're not dishonest.'

Mills' correction was retweeted three times.

It did, however, prompt an apology (sort of) from Shepherd, who wrote: 'I'm going to do the right thing here, with apologies to anyone concerned. There are cranes. I stood where the other photographer (Ben, I believe) stood and the cranes are there. I stand by my original tweet: I'm writing this from the location and I can see no breaching of lockdown.'

But that didn't stop the questions on Twitter. Here's just one of them: 'Jon. The shadows in the picture are <40 per cent of the height of the object. On the day claimed the minimum shadow length would have been 78 per cent of object height? Why the huge discrepancy? To be that short would be close to summer solstice, and before iPhone11 on sale?'

And it still didn't stop the abuse being levelled at the *Daily Express*. This was tweeted the next day: 'I've lived in Brighton and Hove for 6-7 years and have only ever seen the seafront this busy during the height of summer and know for a fact that the sun is never that high in the sky during April I'm calling bullshit on the Daily Express, aka once again more Tory Propaganda.'

The *Mail on Sunday* faced a complaint that it used a photo from 2015 to illustrate a story on the reopening of live meat markets in China. The paper was able to prove the picture was taken on 28 March 2020, as it had reported. It turned out that the complaint was based on wrong information somebody had seen posted online.

The same newspaper was rapped on the knuckles by IPSO

over a columnist's claims that 'a major experiment' showed that masks were 'useless'. The panel found that the study being referred to, DanMask-19, did not find masks to be ineffective in the transmission of COVID, adding: 'Newspapers must take care not to publish inaccurate information, even in comment pieces.'

Ofcom came down hard on a David Icke interview on London Live on 8 April 2020, calling it a 'serious breach' of its regulations after receiving forty-eight complaints from members of the public worried about his 'potentially harmful' statements. It was the usual Icke schtick about a new world order, a 'Hunger Games society' and a ruling cult that wants 'to transform the world economic order into this technocratic, AI-controlled tyranny, and both the Coronavirus and climate change hoax are providing the problem'.

The traditional conformity of the mainstream media explains why it became the biggest bogeyman of the conspiracy theorists during the pandemic. There is a case to be made that it did get left behind in both the speed with which people expected to receive information and the breadth of coverage. The days when people generally believed what they read in their national newspapers and magazines has gone. With so much noise online and computers, tablets and phones delivering updates every few minutes, people aren't waiting to be told what to think.

The pandemic was the new media landscape's first major test in covering a huge, rambling, developing story that impacted just about every person on the planet and it didn't cover itself in glory.

The Russian truth meddlers were ready and so were the so-called conspiracy theorists who jumped on COVID as an opportunity to fast-track their agendas and reach audiences far bigger than previously possible. But such was the level of distrust alluded to by Lee McIntyre in an earlier chapter, that ordinary people just were not prepared to believe everything they were told by their government and their traditional sources of news such as newspapers and TV. Inevitably, they looked to their phones, tablets and computers for answers.

The sense of being all in it together engendered by Captain Sir Tom Moore and his efforts to raise £33 million for the NHS and the Thursday night ovations for frontline workers dissipated in Britain with the stuttering approach of Boris Johnson's government.

In America it was even worse. Fights have broken out in school board meetings, on planes and at council meetings over vaccines and masks. If you ventured into a supermarket without a face covering, you were deemed a Trump-loving Republican. Rather than pulling together in a time of crisis, many countries – the United States being a prime example – were pulled apart by political partisanship that directly impacted the way the pandemic was seen by the public.

For instance, the conservative media in the US initially played down COVID-19, echoing President Donald Trump's stated view that it was little worse than flu, while more left-leaning outlets, perhaps shell-shocked by Trump's bombastic presidency, dismissed some of his administration's claims that should have been given more attention. The lab leak theory, as we have already discussed, was a case in point.

In a live broadcast on 24 October 2021, Jair Bolsonaro, the president of Brazil, claimed vaccines could increase the chance of contracting AIDS. Is it any wonder people didn't know whom to trust?

As COVID-19 variants continued to cut a swathe through the world's populations, coverage was eventually reduced to daily league tables in the UK while the conversations turned to dancers on *Strictly* and Premier League footballers refusing to get vaccinated.

The Reuters Institute at Oxford University published the results of a YouGov survey as part of its 'UK COVID News and Information Project' found that one third (35 per cent) of people polled between 13 and 19 August 2020 said they thought the coronavirus crisis in the UK had been made worse by the way the news media covered it, and just 7 per cent said it had been made better.

A similar poll the previous month put the proportion of the UK population that 'always or often actively avoid the news' at 22 per cent. 'Most COVID-19 news avoiders say that they avoid news on television (77 per cent), followed by news websites/apps (51 per cent), social media (50 per cent), print (48 per cent) and radio (41 per cent),' it adds.

A study published in *The Lancet* in January 2021 shows that media coverage of the pandemic decreased after the initial flurry of attention despite COVID's continued spread. During February and March 2020, the number of stories about COVID in 102 of the high circulation sources across fifty countries rose precipitously but, says the study, 'media coverage has steadily waned since the last week of March, despite the continued rapid and global spread of COVID-19 over the months that followed.'

I am sure that if you ask any anti-vaxxer where they get their news it won't be from the *Daily Mail* or the *Guardian*, for that matter, and it won't be from the BBC or Sky. They will follow people like Piers Robinson, Nick Hudson, Ivor Cummins, Clare Craig, Simone Gold and Dan Astin-Gregory. They will rail against the ways those in power are deplatforming the scientific debate over COVID-19 and the best ways to combat the virus.

And they do have a point.

That's why we need an independent, free speech-biased, First Amendment-supporting body to regulate what is posted online. Not to block debate, just to moderate it.

Let's be clear, the existing bodies are far from perfect.

The *Guardian*, *The Independent* and the *Financial Times* all have major misgivings about IPSO's independence and declined to take part. Their chief complaint is that IPSO's budget is controlled by the Regulatory Funding Company, which is made up of four elected directors from national newspaper publishers, three from the regional press, one from the Scottish press and one from the magazine industry. It also has a say over the make-up of IPSO's twelve-member board. It's worth remembering that about 90 per cent of the UK print media is owned by just three companies, Rupert Murdoch's News UK, Reach PLC (formerly Trinity Mirror) and the *Daily Mail*'s parent group, DMG Media.

Although Ofcom calls itself independent, and is independently financed by the companies it regulates, as a statutory corporation there is a direct connection to the Department for Culture, Media and Sport, where the Secretary of State must present its report each year to the House of Commons. Whether they want to admit it or not, there is pressure from Parliament.

In December 2020, the UK government added 'online harms' to Ofcom's responsibilities, meaning it has now added the internet to its stable. Announcing the move, Ofcom's chief executive Melanie Dawes said that 'being online brings huge benefits, but four in five people have concerns about it. That shows the need for sensible, balanced rules that protect users from serious harm, but also recognise the great things about being online, including free expression.'

Ofcom says most people support tighter rules but adds: 'We won't censor the web or social media. Free expression is the lifeblood of the internet and it's central to our democracy, values and modern society. Our role in upholding broadcasting standards for TV and radio programmes means we've gained extensive experience of protecting audiences from harm while upholding freedom of expression. An important part of our job will be to ensure online platforms do the same with their systems and processes.'

Importantly, however, it adds: 'We won't be responsible for regulating or moderating individual pieces of online content. The Government's intention is that online platforms should have appropriate systems and processes in place to protect the user; and that Ofcom should take action against them if they fall short. We'll focus particular attention on tackling the most serious harms, including illegal content and harms affecting children.'

That suggests to me that Ofcom and the British government isn't taking the challenge that new media represents anything like as seriously as it should. Just to deal with the disinformation being spread purposely and relentlessly by the Russians should be a good enough reason to set up a new overseer.

Create some boundaries, make it fair and, crucially, protect the public. I'm convinced that some independent thinkers who have been deplatformed would return and flourish under a free speech regulator; some others would be banished for good. But the decisions would come from a transparently run body with specialist experts, not random, faceless staffers from Twitter, Facebook and the others. You couldn't be banned from Twitter because Elon Musk isn't a fan – or reinstated because he is.

As for the elephant in the room lab leak conspiracy theory running through the pandemic, that's a simpler study with an even more difficult solution. Most people, governments, scientists, and conspiracy theorists, accept now that the initial outbreak could be the result of a lab leak in China.

The evidence, with all its gaps, is still too seductive to believe anything else. The lack of care over the handling of bats in the wild was an accident waiting to happen and the smokescreen stories about the Wuhan wet market being ground zero lost their lustre after it emerged that no bats were for sale at the time, nor were there any pangolins, the desperate creature saddled wrongly with blame for piggy-backing the virus.

The answers are out there. Bat Woman and Robin, Wuhan's bat virology experts, remain as mysterious as their fictional counterparts and still haven't fully explained what their research entailed in the lead up to the outbreak.

There have been no explanations how or why key data at Wuhan's Institute of Virology went missing and, whatever they say, WHO officials were not given the kind of access they needed for a proper investigation.

There's no evidence that the Chinese were developing a bioweapon – although the concept is not completely implausible – but there is a probability that the bat samples collected after the Yunnan mine outbreak were being worked on in Wuhan and the security over handling of the viruses has certainly been questioned.

From what we know, the bat virus that killed three miners and sickened three others did not spread to villagers living nearby or to medical staff who treated the six men. The Chinese virologists argue that it wasn't even the same SARS-CoV-2 virus. But there are simply too many links, too many coincidences, to ignore. This must be conjecture because key information has still been withheld from investigators, but what if virologists in Wuhan were manipulating the bat virus, quite possibly for altruistic motives, and at a certain point there was a leak of some kind that put that mutated virus into circulation? If this hypothesis turned out to be anything like correct, China would face global condemnation and demands for compensation enough to cripple even the richest country in the world (on pure wealth, China's net worth is $113 trillion compared to second-placed US at $50 trillion, although if you are ranking by GDP per capita, the richest is Luxembourg). Reason enough, you may think, to keep schtum.

Call this a conspiracy theory if you like, but China's secrecy has made it impossible to get to the truth. Questions are being asked – questions should be asked – but we are not getting any answers. The more we know about the dangers of COVID-19 and the effects it is having on our lives, the less 'fake news' the fantasists can spin to derail the truth and, as we have seen, put actual lives in danger. We must know what happened in Wuhan, both to spike the nationalism and to learn from so it can never be allowed to happen again.

The world has been changed for ever by the events of the past few years. It is crucial that history offers an accurate account of what happened.

I'm lucky, my COVID will pass, and my life will carry on. But too many people have died needlessly through the pandemic. We owe it to them to ensure that future generations don't make the same mistakes.

Governments have been too stringent and perhaps too impatient to listen to those with voices raising opinions that conflict with the science they are following. The growing numbers who are distrustful of authority have also lost patience with those in power to the extent that they are willing to play

Russian roulette with their own lives.

There's a balance out there and perhaps it can be found in the very nature of science as something that flows and changes through time as we gain better understanding of all its wonder.

It's vital that we keep our minds open to new possibilities and not closed off to alternative ways of thinking, just as long as no more lives are put at risk as a result.

Science never stands still, and neither should we.

SOURCES

▼

Chapter 1

Study: Analysis of Six Patients With Unknown Viruses, Master's Thesis by Li Xuhttps://www.documentcloud.org/documents/6981198-Analysis-of-Six-Patients-With-Unknown-Viruses.html

The Times: 'Revealed: Seven year coronavirus trail from mine deaths to a Wuhan lab' (Saturday, 4 July 2020) https://www.thetimes.co.uk/article/seven-year-covid-trail-revealed-l5vxt7jqpStudy: Lethal Pneumonia Cases in Mojiang Miners (2012) and the Mineshaft Could Provide Important Clues to the Origin of SARS-CoV-2, Monali C. Rahalkar and Rahul A. Bahulikar https://www.frontiersin.org/articles/10.3389/fpubh.2020.581569/full#B2

Social media: Twitter posts, The Seeker https://twitter.com/TheSeeker268/status/1266279461516763136/photo/1

Wall Street Journal: 'The Wuhan Lab Leak Question: A Disused Chinese Mine Takes Center Stage' (24 May 2021)
https://www.wsj.com/articles/wuhan-lab-leak-question-chinese-mine-covid-pandemic-11621871125

Chapter 2

South China Morning Post: 'Exclusive | Coronavirus: China's first confirmed Covid-19 case traced back to November 17' (13 March 2020)
https://www.scmp.com/news/china/society/article/3074991/coronavirus-chinas-first-confirmed-covid-19-case-traced-backDocument: 'Novel Coronavirus Circulated Undetected Months before First COVID-19 Cases in Wuhan, China', UC San Diego Health (18 March 2021)
https://health.ucsd.edu/news/releases/Pages/2021-03-18-novel-coronavirus-circulated-undetected-months-before-first-covid-19-cases-in-wuhan-china.aspx

Daily Mail: 'What it's REALLY like to catch coronavirus: First British victim, 25, describes how "worst disease he ever had" left him sweating, shivering, and struggling to breathe as his eyes burned and bones ached' (4 March 2020)
https://www.dailymail.co.uk/news/article-8075633/First-British-victim-25-describes-coronavirus.html

Chapter 3

Scientific American: 'How China's "Bat Woman" Hunted Down Viruses from SARS to the New Coronavirus' (1 June 2020)
https://www.scientificamerican.com/article/how-chinas-bat-woman-hunted-down-viruses-from-sars-to-the-new-coronavirus1/

Research article: 'Coexistence of multiple coronaviruses in several bat colonies in an abandoned mineshaft' Research article (18 February 2016) https://link.springer.com/article/10.1007/s12250-016-3713-9

Chapter 4
Washington Post: 'A scientist adventurer and China's "Bat Woman" are under scrutiny as coronavirus lab-leak theory gets another look' (3 June 2021)
https://www.washingtonpost.com/world/asia_pacific/coronavirus-bats-china-wuhan/2021/06/02/772ef984-beb2-11eb-922a-c40c9774bc48_story.html
Wuhan Evening News: 'The post-80s "disease control" guy caught tens of thousands of insects every night to watch cockroaches for research' (3 May 2017)
http://www.xinhuanet.com//local/2017-05/03/c_1120909064_2.htm

Daily Mail: 'Documentary showing a Chinese virus researcher catching wild bats inside Hubei caves fuels conspiracy theory that the coronavirus may have originated in Wuhan's CDC' (1 April 2020)
https://www.dailymail.co.uk/news/article-8172891/Documentary-Wuhan-virologist-catching-wild-bats-fuels-conspiracy-theory.html

Washington Times: 'China researchers isolated bat coronaviruses near Wuhan wild animal market' (30 March 2020)
https://www.washingtontimes.com/news/2020/mar/30/china-researchers-isolated-bat-coronaviruses-near-/

Video: Youth in the Wilderness – Invisible Defense Line, China Science Communication
http://video-old.kepuchina.cn/qt/content_36762.shtml

Document: 'WHO-convened global study of origins of SARS-CoV-2: China Part', WHO Report (14 January–10 February 2021)
https://www.who.int/publications/i/item/who-convened-global-study-of-origins-of-sars-cov-2-china-part

Chapter 5
The Lancet: Study: Genomic characterization and epidemiology of 2019 novel coronavirus: implications for virus origins and receptor binding (30 January 2020)
https://www.thelancet.com/article/S0140-6736(20)30251-8/fulltext

The Conversation: 'What is the ACE2 receptor, how is it connected to coronavirus and why might it be key to treating COVID-19? The experts explain' (14 May 2020)
https://theconversation.com/what-is-the-ace2-receptor-how-is-it-connected-to-coronavirus-and-why-might-it-be-key-to-treating-covid-19-the-experts-explain-136928

Nature.com: Animal sales from Wuhan wet markets immediately prior to the COVID-19 pandemic (Pictures) (7 June 2021)
https://www.nature.com/articles/s41598-021-91470-2

Oxford University Science Blog: 'The wet market sources of Covid-19: bats and pangolins have an alibi' (7 June 2021)https://www.ox.ac.uk/news/science-blog/wet-market-sources-covid-19-bats-and-pangolins-have-alibi

The New Yorker: 'Did Pangolin Trafficking Cause the Coronavirus Pandemic?' (31 August 2020)
https://www.newyorker.com/magazine/2020/08/31/did-pangolins-start-the-coronavirus-pandemic

Nature.com: 'Mystery deepens over animal source of coronavirus' (26 February 2020)https://www.nature.com/articles/d41586-020-00548-w

New York Times: 'Pangolins Are Suspected as a Potential Coronavirus Host' (10 February 2020)https://www.nytimes.com/2020/02/10/science/pangolin-coronavirus.html

Chapter 6

Study: The Possible Origins of 2019-nCoV Coronavirus (February 2020)
https://img-prod.tgcom24.mediaset.it images/2020/02/16/114720192-5eb8307f-017c-4075-a697-348628da0204.pdf

MIT Technology Review: 'Meet the scientist at the center of the covid lab leak controversy' (9 February 2022)
https://www.technologyreview.com/2022/02/09/1044985/shi-zhengli-covid-lab-leak-wuhan/

Wall Street Journal: 'Coronavirus Epidemic Draws Scrutiny to Labs Handling Deadly Pathogens' (5 March 2020)
https://www.wsj.com/articles/coronavirus-epidemic-draws-scrutiny-to-labs-handling-deadly-pathogens-11583349777

Chapter 7

BBC: 'How smallpox claimed its final victim' (10 August 2018)
https://www.bbc.com/news/uk-england-birmingham-45101091

Mother Jones: 'The Non-Paranoid Person's Guide to Viruses
Escaping From Labs' (14 May 2020)
https://www.motherjones.com/politics/2020/05/the-non-paranoid-
persons-guide-to-viruses-escaping-from-labs/

Bloomberg: 'The History of Lab Leaks Has Lots of Entries' (27 May
2021)
https://www.bloomberg.com/opinion/articles/2021-05-27/covid-
19-and-lab-leak-history-smallpox-h1n1-sars

New York Times: 'Where Did the Coronavirus Come From? What
We Already Know Is Troubling' (25 June 2021)
https://www.nytimes.com/2021/06/25/opinion/coronavirus-lab.
html

Document: The Cambridge Working Group, Statement (14 July
2014)
http://www.cambridgeworkinggroup.org/

Newsweek: 'The Controversial Experiments and Wuhan Lab
Suspected of Starting the Coronavirus Pandemic' (27 March 2020)
https://www.newsweek.com/controversial-wuhan-
lab-experiments-that-may-have-started-coronavirus-
pandemic-1500503

Chapter 8

Washington Post: 'Tom Cotton keeps repeating a coronavirus fringe theory that scientists have disputed' (17 February 2020) https://www.washingtonpost.com/politics/2020/02/16/tom-cotton-coronavirus-conspiracy/

Washington Post: 'Experts debunk fringe theory linking China's coronavirus to weapons research' (29 January 2020) https://www.washingtonpost.com/world/2020/01/29/experts-debunk-fringe-theory-linking-chinas-coronavirus-weapons-research/

The Hill: 'Tom Cotton once again makes media look foolish' (30 May 2021) https://thehill.com/opinion/healthcare/556056-tom-cotton-once-again-makes-media-look-foolish?rl=1

BBC.com: 'Coronavirus: Trump stands by China lab origin theory for virus' (1 May 2020) https://www.bbc.com/news/world-us-canada-52496098

Time: 'How Distrust of Donald Trump Muddled the COVID-19 "Lab Leak" Debate' (26 May 2021) https://time.com/6051414/donald-trump-wuhan-laboratory-leak/

Chapter 9

CNN/
YouTube: She's the target of a coronavirus conspiracy theory. Now she's afraid for her life https://www.youtube.com/watch?v=qXJJYBb-kzw

CNN Business: 'Exclusive: She's been falsely accused of starting the pandemic. Her life has been turned upside down' (27 April 2020) https://www.cnn.com/2020/04/27/tech/coronavirus-conspiracy-theory/index.html

New York Times: 'Deadly Germ Research Is Shut Down at Army Lab Over Safety Concerns' (5 August 2019) https://www.nytimes.com/2019/08/05/health/germs-fort-detrick-biohazard.html
Department of Defense News: 'US Women Place 8th Despite Crash in 50-Mile Cycling Race' (25 October 2019) https://www.defense.gov/News/News-Stories/Article/Article/1998827/us-women-place-8th-despite-crash-in-50-mile-cycling-race/
Army Times: 'Conspiracies falsely accuse an Army reservist of being "patient zero" of coronavirus pandemic' (28 April 2020) https://www.armytimes.com/news/your-army/2020/04/28/conspiracies-falsely-accuse-an-army-reservist-of-being-patient-zero-of-coronavirus-pandemic/CNN: 'Chinese diplomat promotes conspiracy theory that US military brought coronavirus to Wuhan' (13 March 2020) https://www.cnn.com/2020/03/13/asia/china-coronavirus-us-lijian-zhao-intl-hnk/index.html

Social media: Tweet, Li Yang, Counsellor of Department of Information, MFA, China, Former Consul General of China in Rio de Janeiro (28 June 2021) https://twitter.com/Li_Yang_China/status/1409748169261518851

Foreign Policy: 'China Fires Back at Biden With Conspiracy Theories About Maryland Lab' (9 July 2021)

https://foreignpolicy.com/2021/07/09/china-fires-back-at-biden-with-conspiracy-theories-about-maryland-lab/

NBC News: 'China-linked disinformation campaign blames Covid on Maine lobsters' (21 October 2021)
https://www.nbcnews.com/news/china-linked-disinformation-campaign-blames-covid-maine-lobsters-rcna3236

Chapter 10
Wall Street Journal: 'Intelligence on Sick Staff at Wuhan Lab Fuels Debate on Covid-19 Origin' (23 May 2021)
https://www.wsj.com/articles/intelligence-on-sick-staff-at-wuhan-lab-fuels-debate-on-covid-19-origin-11621796228
Document: Statement by President Joe Biden on the Investigation into the Origins of COVID-19 (26 May 2021)
https://www.whitehouse.gov/briefing-room/statements-releases/2021/05/26/statement-by-president-joe-biden-on-the-investigation-into-the-origins-of-covid-19/
BBC.com: 'Covid: Biden orders investigation into virus origin as lab leak theory debated' (27 May 2021)
https://www.bbc.com/news/world-us-canada-57260009

Vanity Fair: 'The Lab-Leak Theory: Inside the Fight to Uncover COVID-19's Origins' (3 June 2021)
https://www.vanityfair.com/news/2021/06/the-lab-leak-theory-inside-the-fight-to-uncover-covid-19s-origins

New York Post: 'Trump proclaims "I was right" as HHS chief urges WHO probe into Wuhan "lab leak"' (25 May 2021)
https://nypost.com/2021/05/25/hhs-secretary-xavier-becerra-urges-who-to-launch-new-covid-probe/

New York Times: 'New Research Points to Wuhan Market as Pandemic Origin' (26 February 2022)
https://www.nytimes.com/interactive/2022/02/26/science/covid-virus-wuhan-origins.html?referringSource=articleShare

Chapter 11
YouTube: 'Gove warns 5G-coronavirus conspiracy theory is "dangerous nonsense"', Video (4 April 2020)
https://www.youtube.com/watch?v=uf2HpbDCM9I

Social media: Tweet, Charlie Haynes
https://twitter.com/charliehtweets/
status/1245722007947411458?ref_src=twsrc per cent5Etfw per cent7Ctwcamp per cent5Etweetembed per cent7Ctwterm per cent5E1245722007947411458 per cent7Ctwgr per cent5E per cent7Ctwcon per cent5Es1_&ref_url=https per cent3A per cent2F per cent2Fwww.gq.com per cent2Fstory per cent2Fcoronavirus-5g-conspiracy-theory-explained

Observer: 'The inconvenient truth about cancer and mobile phones' (14 July 2018)
https://www.theguardian.com/technology/2018/jul/14/mobile-phones-cancer-inconvenient-truths

Observer: 'Mobile phones and cancer – the full picture' (21 July 2018)
https://www.theguardian.com/technology/2018/jul/21/mobile-phones-are-not-a-health-hazard

New York Times: 'Your 5G Phone Won't Hurt You. But Russia Wants You to Think Otherwise' (12 May 2019)
https://www.nytimes.com/2019/05/12/
science/5g-phone-safety-health-russia.
html?action=click&module=RelatedLinks&pgtype=Article

GQ.com: 'Here's the Bonkers Conspiracy Theory Blaming 5G for the Coronavirus' (7 April 2020)
https://www.gq.com/story/coronavirus-5g-conspiracy-theory-explained

Huffington Post: 'No, Keri Hilson, 5G Did Not Cause Coronavirus' (6 April 2020)
https://www.huffpost.com/entry/keri-hilson-5g-did-not-cause-cor
onavirus_n_5e6f8ba7c5b6dda30fce0348

Chapter 12

BBC.com: 'Coronavirus: Outcry after Trump suggests injecting disinfectant as treatment' (24 April 2020)
https://www.bbc.com/news/world-us-canada-52407177

Document: 'Danger: Don't Drink Miracle Mineral Solution or Similar Products', US Food and Drug Administration website
https://www.fda.gov/consumers/consumer-updates/danger-dont-drink-miracle-mineral-solution-or-similar-products

New York Times: 'Small Chloroquine Study Halted Over Risk of Fatal Heart Complications' (12 April 2020)
https://www.nytimes.com/2020/04/12/health/chloroquine-coronavirus-trump.html

Science: '"This is insane!"' Many scientists lament Trump's embrace of risky malaria drugs for coronavirus' (26 March 2020) https://www.science.org/content/article/insane-many-scientists-lament-trump-s-embrace-risky-malaria-drugs-coronavirus

BuzzFeed News: 'Trump Gets Very Angry When People Talk About The Virus That's Killed 225,000 In The US' (26 October 2020) https://www.buzzfeednews.com/article/kadiagoba/coronavirus-donald-trump-covid

Chapter 13

Document: 'Arizona Man Sentenced to 41 Months in Prison On Felony Charge in Jan. 6 Capitol Breach', U.S . District Attorney's Office, District of Columbia, Press Release (17 November 2021) https://www.justice.gov/usao-dc/pr/arizona-man-sentenced-41-months-prison-felony-charge-jan-6-capitol-breach

Guardian: 'One in four Britons believe in QAnon-linked theories', survey (21 October 2020) https://www.theguardian.com/us-news/2020/oct/22/one-in-four-britons-believe-in-qanon-linked-theories-survey

BBC.com: 'What's behind the rise of QAnon in the UK?' (13 October 2020) https://www.bbc.com/news/blogs-trending-54065470

Politico: 'QAnon goes European' (23 October 2020) https://www.politico.eu/article/qanon-europe-coronavirus-protests/

New York Times: 'What Is QAnon, the Viral Pro-Trump Conspiracy Theory?' (21 September 2021)
https://www.nytimes.com/article/what-is-qanon.html

Nature.com: 'Tracking QAnon: how Trump turned conspiracy-theory research upside down' (4 February 2021)
https://www.nature.com/articles/d41586-021-00257-y

Chapter 14

Website: The DRASTIC A Team
https://drasticresearch.org/the-team/

Newsweek: 'Exclusive: How Amateur Sleuths Broke the Wuhan Lab Story and Embarrassed the Media' (2 June 2021)
https://www.newsweek.com/exclusive-how-amateur-sleuths-broke-wuhan-lab-story-embarrassed-media-1596958

Wall Street Journal: WHO Investigators to Scrap Plans for Interim Report on Probe of Covid-19 Origins (5 March 2021)
https://www.wsj.com/articles/who-investigators-to-scrap-interim-report-on-probe-of-covid-19-origins-11614865067

Document: Open Letter to the WHO COVID-19 International Investigation Team (March 2021)
https://www.ipetitions.com/petition/open-letter-to-the-who-covid-19-international

Document: Call for a Full and Unrestricted International Forensic Investigation into the Origins of COVID-19, Letter (4 March 2021)
https://s.wsj.net/public/resources/documents/COVID per cent20OPEN per cent20LETTER per cent20FINAL per cent20030421 per cent20(1).pdf

Wall Street Journal: 'In new documentary, WHO scientist says Chinese officials pressured investigation to drop lab-leak hypothesis' (12 August 2021)
https://www.washingtonpost.com/world/2021/08/12/who-origins-embarek/

Social media: Looking for Wilson Edwards, Tweet, Swiss Embassy in Beijing
https://twitter.com/SwissEmbChina/status/1425042973289504770

Chapter 15
Science: 'Biocompatible near-infrared quantum dots delivered to the skin by microneedle patches record vaccination' (18 December 2019)
https://www.science.org/doi/10.1126/scitranslmed.aay7162

Social media: Facebook Post: https://www.facebook.com/sam.powell.739/posts/3078281155543083

USA Today: 'Fact check: Bill Gates is not planning to microchip the world through a COVID-19 vaccine' (20 June 2020)
https://www.usatoday.com/story/news/factcheck/2020/06/12/fact-check-bill-gates-isnt-planning-implant-microchips-via-vaccines/3171405001/

ABC4: 'No, COVID-19 vaccine patients are not being injected with a microchip' (8 February 2021) https://www.abc4.com/news/digital-exclusives/no-covid-19-vaccine-patients-are-not-being-injected-with-a-microchip/

Blog: '31 questions and answers about COVID-19', Gates Notes (19 March 2020) https://www.gatesnotes.com/Health/A-coronavirus-AMA

Daily Mail: 'Bill Gates says he's shocked by "crazy and evil" conspiracy theories linking him to COVID-19 including claims he wanted to use vaccines to microchip billions' (27 January 2021) https://www.dailymail.co.uk/news/article-9192815/Bill-Gates-says-hes-shocked-crazy-evil-conspiracy-theories-linking-COVID-19.html

Chapter 16
Website: The Great Reset, Prince Charles Home Page (3 June 2020) https://www.princeofwales.gov.uk/thegreatreset

Social media: Prince Charles Tweet (3 June 2020) https://twitter.com/ClarenceHouse/status/1268189467959070733?ref_src=twsrc per cent5Etfw per cent7Ctwcamp per cent5Etweetembed per cent7Ctwterm per cent5E1268189467959070733 per cent7Ctwgr per cent5E per cent7Ctwcon per cent5Es1_&ref_url=https per cent3A per cent2F per cent2Fwww.princeofwales.gov.uk per cent2Fthegreatreset

YouTube: The Great Reset, Royal Family Page, Video (3 June 2020)https://www.youtube.com/watch?v=hRPQqfwwuhU

WE Forum: 'Now is the time for a 'great reset', Klaus Schwab, Video
(3 June 2020)
https://www.weforum.org/agenda/2020/06/now-is-the-time-for-a-great-reset

Document: Open Letter to the President of the United States of America
Donald J. Trump, Archbishop Carlo Maria Viganò (25 October 2020)
https://catholicfamilynews.com/blog/2020/10/30/open-letter-to-president-donald-trump/

Fox News: Laura Ingraham – The Angle, Video (13 November 2020)
https://video.foxnews.com/v/6209546305001#sp=show-clips

Fox News: Tucker Carlson – 'The elites want COVID-19 lockdowns to usher in a "Great Reset" and that should terrify you' (16 November 2020)
https://www.foxnews.com/opinion/tucker-carlson-coronavirus-pandemic-lockdowns-great-reset

YouTube: Russell Brand – 'WHAT?! The Great Reset Is NOT a Conspiracy!' (30 January 2022)
https://www.youtube.com/watch?v=BXTPzFSx6oI

Social media: '8 predictions for the world in 2030', WEF Facebook (18 November 2016)
https://www.facebook.com/worldeconomicforum/videos/8-predictions-for-the-world-in-2030/10153982130966479/

Chapter 17

BBC.com: 'Coronavirus: How my mum became a conspiracy theory influencer' (26 October 2021)
https://www.bbc.com/news/av/uk-54669239

Document: Nursing and Midwifery Council Fitness to Practise Committee (26–28 May 2021)
https://www.nmc.org.uk/globalassets/sitedocuments/ftpoutcomes/2021/may-2021/reasons-shemirani-ftpcsm-76998-20210528.pdf

Social media: Twitter, Sebastian Shemirani (16 July 2021)
https://twitter.com/BBCr4today/status/1419599993124671488?ref_src=twsrc per cent5Etfw per cent7Ctwcamp per cent5Etweetembed per cent7Ctwterm per cent5E1419599993124671488 per cent7Ctwgr per cent5E per cent7Ctwcon per cent5Es1_&ref_url=https per cent3A per cent2F per cent2Fnypost.com per cent2F2021 per cent2F07 per cent2F26 per cent2Fson-of-covid-conspiracy-theorist-says-mom-should-be-prosecuted per cent2F

New York Times: 'Marjorie Taylor Greene reportedly endorsed executing Democrats on Facebook before she was elected to Congress' (27 January 2021)
https://www.nytimes.com/2021/01/27/us/marjorie-taylor-greene-executing-democrats.html

Chapter 18

Document: The Vaccine Death Report (September 2021)
https://indepthnh.org/wp-content/uploads/2021/10/COVID-Report-from-Rep.-Weyler-3.pdf

Document: Information for UK recipients on COVID-19 Vaccine AstraZeneca (Regulation 174)
https://www.gov.uk/government/publications/regulatory-approval-of-covid-19-vaccine-astrazeneca/information-for-uk-recipients-on-covid-19-vaccine-astrazeneca
Document: Information for UK recipients on Pfizer/BioNTech COVID-19 vaccine (Regulation 174)
https://www.gov.uk/government/publications/regulatory-approval-of-pfizer-biontech-vaccine-for-covid-19/information-for-uk-recipients-on-pfizerbiontech-covid-19-vaccine

Website: Vaccine Knowledge Project, University of Oxford
https://vk.ovg.ox.ac.uk/vk/covid-19-vaccines

Guardian: '"They're building a massive lasagne": man behind WhatsApp virus spoof revealed' (21 March 2020)
https://www.theguardian.com/technology/2020/mar/21/a-lasagne-the-size-of-wembley-whatsapp-joke-swallowed-whole

Reuters: 'False claim: Putin released lions on the streets of Russia to enforce coronavirus lockdown' (25 March 2020)
https://www.reuters.com/article/uk-factcheck-putin-lions-coronavirus-loc/false-claim-putin-released-lions-on-the-streets-of-russia-to-enforce-coronavirus-lockdown-idUSKBN21C371

Document: 'The use of cow dung and urine to cure COVID-19 in India: A public health concern' (26 May 2021)
https://onlinelibrary.wiley.com/doi/full/10.1002/hpm.3257

Chapter 19

Document: 'How Big Tech powers and profits from David Icke's lies and hate, and why it must stop'
https://www.counterhate.com/_files/ugd/f4d9b9_
db8ff469f6914534ac02309bb488f948.pdf

Chapter 20

Website: https://www.pandata.org/about/

YouTube: Interview: President Barack Obama, Video (6 April 2022)
https://www.youtube.com/watch?v=guO3_7pn7FI

Chapter 21

Document: 'The Disinformation Dozen', Center for Countering Digital Hate
https://www.counterhate.com/_files/ugd/f4d9b9_
b7cedc0553604720b7137f8663366ee5.pdf

Social media: RFK JR on Alec Baldwin Show, Instagram
https://www.instagram.com/p/CDjp_xdl7wG/?utm_source=ig_
embed&utm_campaign=embed_video_watch_again

New York Times: 'The Most Influential Spreader of Coronavirus Misinformation Online' (24 July 2021)
https://www.nytimes.com/2021/07/24/technology/joseph-mercola-
coronavirus-misinformation-online.html

Chapter 22
Newsweek: 'Flat Earthers, and the Rise of Science Denial in America' (14 May 2019)
https://www.newsweek.com/flat-earth-science-denial-america-1421936

Document: 'How to Spot COVID-19 Conspiracy Theories' (May 2020)
https://www.climatechangecommunication.org/wp-content/uploads/2020/05/How-to-Spot-COVID-19-Conspiracy-Theories.pdf

Website: CIRCE, the Cognitive Immunology Research Collaborative
https://cognitiveimmunology.net/about-circe

Deseret News: 'How the White House "prebunked" Putin's lies' (3 March 2022)
https://www.deseret.com/opinion/2022/3/2/22955870/opinion-how-the-white-house-prebunked-putins-lies-disinformation-joe-biden-donald-trump-russia?fbclid=IwAR3fL8mM5M2D66TswqYxRLhQ9BLBeLBrBEiqwNTC7zmZeymLBUru_Omfl5I

Chapter 23
Oriental Review: 'Bill Gates, Vaccinations, Microchips, And Patent 060606' (29 April 2020)
https://orientalreview.org/2020/04/29/bill-gates-vaccinations-microchips-and-patent-060606/comment-page-1/

Document: Top of Form

Bottom of Form

Top of Form

'WO2020060606 – Cryptocurrency System Using Body Activity Data'

https://patentscope.wipo.int/search/en/detail.
jsf?docId=WO2020060606&tab=PCTCLAIMSBottom of Form

Document: 'Pillars of Russia's Disinformation and Propaganda Ecosystem', US Department of State, GEC Special Report (August 2020)

https://www.state.gov/wp-content/uploads/2020/08/Pillars-of-Russia per centE2 per cent80 per cent99s-Disinformation-and-Propaganda-Ecosystem_08-04-20.pdf

Document: 'Treasury Sanctions Russians Bankrolling Putin and Russia-Backed Influence Actors', US Department of Treasury (3 March 2022)

https://home.treasury.gov/news/press-releases/jy0628

Document: Statement of Lea Gabrielle Special Envoy & Coordinator for the Global Engagement Center, US Department of Statehttps://www.foreign.senate.gov/imo/media/doc/030520_Gabrielle_Testimony.pdf

New York Times: 'Putin's Long War Against American Science' (13 April 2020)

https://www.nytimes.com/2020/04/13/science/putin-russia-disinformation-health-coronavirus.html

Chapter 24

Social media: Twitter, Nicki Minaj
https://twitter.com/NICKIMINAJ/
status/1437532566945341441?s=20

Social media: Twitter, Nicki Minaj
https://twitter.com/NICKIMINAJ/
status/1437526877808128000?s=20

Guardian: 'Nicki Minaj claim that Covid vaccine can cause
impotence dismissed by Trinidad and Tobago' 15 September 2021
https://www.theguardian.com/world/2021/sep/15/nicki-minaj-
covid-vaccine-claim-impotence-dismissed-trinidad-and-tobago

UKHSA: 'Latest data reinforces the safety of COVID-19
vaccinations in pregnant women' (27 January 2022)
https://www.gov.uk/government/news/latest-data-reinforces-the-
safety-of-covid-19-vaccinations-in-pregnant-women

NHS: 'Unvaccinated mothers share harrowing stories to urge
pregnant women to get jabbed', Video (4 December 2021)
https://www.youtube.com/watch?v=024covX-d9M&t=247s

Manchester Evening News: 'Unvaccinated pregnant women make
up nearly a fifth of the worst recent Covid cases' (11 October 2021)
https://www.manchestereveningnews.co.uk/news/uk-news/
unvaccinated-pregnant-women-make-up-21821430

NBC News: '"Misinformation killed her": Bride-to-be who hesitated to get vaccinated dies of Covid' (15 September 2021)
https://www.nbcnews.com/news/us-news/misinformation-killed-her-bride-be-who-hesitated-get-vaccinated-dies-n1279263

Chapter 25
Document: The Great Barrington Declaration (2–4 October 2020)
https://gbdeclaration.org/#read
Social media: Twitter, Gregg Gonsalves
https://twitter.com/gregggonsalves/status/1313188071937060870

Guardian: 'Scientists call for Covid herd immunity strategy for young' (5 October 2020)
https://www.theguardian.com/world/2020/oct/06/scientists-call-for-herd-immunity-covid-strategy-for-young

The Spectator: 'Why can't we talk about the Great Barrington Declaration?' (17 October 2020)
https://www.spectator.co.uk/article/why-cant-we-talk-about-the-great-barrington-declaration

Website: World Doctors Alliance
https://worlddoctorsalliance.com/about/

Document: 'Focused Protection: The Middle Ground between Lockdowns and "Let it Rip"' (25 November 2020)
https://gbdeclaration.org/focused-protection/

Chapter 26

GRFTR: 'Why Was a Major Study on Ivermectin for COVID-19 Just Retracted?' (15 July 2021)
https://grftr.news/why-was-a-major-study-on-ivermectin-for-covid-19-just-retracted/

BuzzFeed News: 'A Prominent Study Said Ivermectin Prevents COVID, But The Data Is Suspect' (27 September 2021)
https://www.buzzfeednews.com/article/stephaniemlee/ivermectin-covid-study-suspect-data

Medium: 'Is Ivermectin for Covid-19 Based on Fraudulent Research?', Blog (15 July 2021)
https://gidmk.medium.com/is-ivermectin-for-covid-19-based-on-fraudulent-research-5cc079278602

Guardian: 'Huge study supporting ivermectin as Covid treatment withdrawn over ethical concerns' (15 July 2021)
https://www.theguardian.com/science/2021/jul/16/huge-study-supporting-ivermectin-as-covid-treatment-withdrawn-over-ethical-concerns

US Food & Drug Administration: 'Why You Should Not Use Ivermectin to Treat or Prevent COVID-19', Document (12 October 2021)
https://www.fda.gov/consumers/consumer-updates/why-you-should-not-use-ivermectin-treat-or-prevent-covid-19

Social media: Twitter, FDA, 'You are not a horse. You are not a cow. Seriously, y'all. Stop it.'
https://twitter.com/US_FDA/status/1429050070243192839?ref_src=twsrc per cent5Etfw

BBC: 'Ivermectin: How false science created a Covid "miracle" drug' (6 October 2021)
https://www.bbc.co.uk/news/health-58170809

YouTube: 'Dr Pierre Kory Talks About Human Rights and The Big Science Disinformation', Video (5 May 2021)
https://www.youtube.com/watch?v=LkIKCbwBcLU

ABC News: 'Jim Bakker, his church settle lawsuit over COVID-19 claims' (24 June 2021)
https://abcnews.go.com/Entertainment/wireStory/jim-bakker-church-settle-lawsuit-covid-19-claims-78443031

Chapter 27

The Lancet:
'COVID-19 media coverage decreasing despite deepening crisis' (January 2021)https://www.thelancet.com/journals/lanplh/article/PIIS2542-5196(20)30303-X/fulltext

The Reuters Institute: 'The UK COVID-19 news and information project'
https://reutersinstitute.politics.ox.ac.uk/UK-COVID-19-news-and-information-project

Ofcom: 'Ofcom to regulate harmful content online' (15 December 2020)
https://www.ofcom.org.uk/about-ofcom/latest/features-and-news/ofcom-to-regulate-harmful-content-online

Social media: Twitter, Brighton Seafront (26 April 2020)
https://twitter.com/jonmillsphoto/
status/1254704201256579072?ref_src=twsrc per cent5Etfw

Press Gazette: 'Independent Press Standards Organisation is not independent, but it is probably the best solution we are going to get' (15 November 2013)
https://pressgazette.co.uk/independent-press-standards-organisation-is-not-independent-but-it-is-probably-the-best-solution-we-are-going-to-get

IPSO: The Covid Report 2020/2021
https://www.ipso.co.uk/media/2147/covid-report.pdf

ACKNOWLEDGEMENTS

I would like to offer my heartfelt thanks to Toby Buchan and the team at John Blake Publishing. As always, it has been an absolute pleasure working with Toby. I would also like to thank all the people who contributed to this book. Conspiracy theorists get a bad rap and sometimes for good reason; they can have their own nefarious motives and agendas. But I am grateful to those who were prepared to stand up and say publicly what they genuinely believe to be true with the purer motives of helping others and exposing hypocrisy.

ABOUT THE AUTHOR

David Gardner is a best-selling author and journalist, who worked as an editor with *Newsweek* until 2021. He also worked for the *Daily Mail* as a crime writer and senior foreign correspondent, filing dispatches from war-torn Beirut, covering the first Gulf War – he was the first British print journalist into Baghdad – and travelling around the world on assignments for the award-winning newspaper. He moved to California as the *Mail*'s Los Angeles correspondent, which saw him cover four presidential elections and all the biggest US stories of the past two decades and worked until recently as the London Evening Standard's US correspondent. His most recent book, *9/11: The Conspiracy Theories* was a *Sunday Times* bestseller. His other books include *The Last of the Hitlers* (2001), an account of how he discovered the descendants of the German dictator, *The Tom Hanks Enigma* (John Blake Publishing, 2007) and *Legends: Murder, Lies and Cover-Ups* (John Blake Publishing, 2016), in which he investigated some of the most famous celebrity deaths in recent history, including those of President John F. Kennedy, Marilyn Monroe and Diana, Princess of Wales. He has also written two novels. He divides his time between the UK and LA.